The Badass Life

ALSO BY CHRISTMAS ABBOTT

The Badass Body Diet

The Badass Life

30
AMAZING DAYS TO A LIFETIME OF GREAT HABITS— BODY, MIND, AND SPIRIT

CHRISTMAS ABBOTT

WM

WILLIAM MORROW

An Imprint of HarpercollinsPublishers

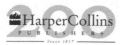

HarperCollins books may be purchased for educational, business, or sales promotional use. For information please e-mail the Special Markets Department at SPsales@harpercollins .com.

FIRST EDITION

Photography by Chloe Crespi.
Meridian illustrations and Inner Smile illustrations courtesy of Lauri Nemetz.
Designed by Bonni Leon-Berman

Library of Congress Cataloging-in-Publication Data has been applied for.

ISBN 978-0-06-264519-7

17 18 19 20 21   LSC   10 9 8 7 6 5 4 3 2 1

This book is dedicated to my two grandmothers, Granny Abbott and my late Grandma Rowland, two women who thrived through discipline, hard work, and standing their ground. Each of you gave me a different understanding of the world and what it meant to be strong in my own way.

GRANNY ABBOTT, you are always the quiet, poised woman but one all the children knew not to cross. Levity and creativity has always flowed through you, which helped me tap into my own creativity. I love hearing your sweet giggle and seeing that bright smile whenever I visit.

GRANDMA ROWLAND, you were the original petite powerhouse. Your fiery sass and aggressively blunt approach helped me discover my own "take me as I am" attitude. You were taken from this world far too soon. Rest in peace, Grandma.

Contents

Introduction

THERE'S A BADASS hiding inside you. It's time to unleash it. I'm not talking about someone who's mean and nasty or a troublemaker. I'm talking about a mentally tough person with a powerfully positive attitude . . . someone who exudes a daring, knowledgeable, make-it-happen drive, with kick-ass charisma . . . someone who pushes the limits in life from all aspects and knows exactly who she is . . . someone who respects mind, body, and spirit and rocks with confidence as a result. When people like this do something—at work, at home, in the gym, wherever they do it *all out*.

The reason this breed of ballsy folks is so successful: They know how to kick bad habits to the curb—and they've done it. I'm talking about bad habits like overeating, not exercising, smoking, abusing alcohol and drugs, and just plain being unkind to yourself. Bad habits mess with your life in a zillion little ways—screwing with your psyche, chipping away at your self-esteem, or putting you at risk of serious physical or mental problems. Consider smoking, for example. It's no secret that this bad habit can ultimately do deadly damage through a heart attack, cancer, or emphysema. So you definitely don't want any bad habits to stall your happiness and success.

How do habits form, anyway? Understand that *we are what we repeatedly do*. If you do something over and over again, the brain cells involved in that behavior begin to sprout tiny fibers called dendrites. With enough repetition of the behavior, those dendrites grow and entwine with other brain cells. Once they're all linked up, your brain has formed a physical circuit called a *neural pathway*, which quickly and efficiently enables the behavior. The new behavior is wired into your brain and is now a habit.

How long does the habit formation process take? It depends on how many times you repeat the behavior. If you repeat it occasionally—like having one or two cock-tails a week—then it's not likely that you'll develop a drinking habit. If you repeat the behavior five or six times a day, and you get some sort of pleasure-producing reward from it, the habit gets ingrained faster, maybe in a month or so. This goes for bad habits as well as good.

What I'm here to help you do is get rid of bad habits and form new ones. And I know all about how to do it. For those of you who don't know me, I'm a fitness trainer, competitive CrossFit athlete, business owner, author, and public speaker, among other things. But I wasn't always this productive. Not at all! From age thirteen until my early twenties, I was a mess, physically and emotionally. I was crazy—and killing myself with my crazy. I was a heavy smoker. I was a druggie. Booze. Meth. Really bad stuff. I couldn't change; I didn't want to change.

So . . . habits, really bad habits? Yes, I know more than a thing or two about how to rid your life of them and be a success. It took me a long time to clear up the wreckage of my life, but through it all, I discovered that buried within my psyche was a mental toughness I didn't know I had. Mental toughness encompasses a lot of qualities. Preparation. Focus. An attitude that drives you to persist and strive for things you consider worthwhile. It's a get-off-your-butt-and-do-something reaction to failure. It's about encouraging thoughts that lead to positive emotions and min-imizing the negative emotions that demotivate you. It's a head game that lets you take absolute control over your life. It's what having a badass life is all about.

You're not born with mental toughness; it's something you develop—which is what this book is all about. Each chapter covers ways to develop mental toughness so you can be the best for yourself. These are action-oriented techniques I've used in my life for years—and techniques I now teach my clients and cover in my sem-inars and speeches: goal setting, self-love, overcoming failures and setbacks, har-nessing positive thinking to attract success, and other issues that will help you seek what makes you happy. All of this is based on my personal experience of creating a better life for myself.

With my own lifestyle and habit shifts, I was able to create a whole new world for myself—a world that I loved and thrived in. I moved up quickly in my work. I was able to create solid business plans with no previous business experience. I implemented practices and created programs that educated, elevated, and empowered my staff. I created nutrition seminars that are uniquely mine—and which would lead to my first book and many additional opportunities.

You can do whatever you want by applying my techniques. You can become more financially secure if you want to. You can become physically fit. You can build a business. You can be more successful in your career and in your relationships. You can find happiness and create a self-fulfilling life. I've seen my personal training clients transformed—not only physically but mentally and spiritually as well—by putting these techniques in play in their lives.

So are you ready to form life-affirming habits, such as mental toughness? Will you push fear out of the picture and take control of your life? Will you give up nasty lifestyle habits that are standing in your way of happiness? Will you get rid of self-limiting thoughts and start living life to the max?

To do all this, you have to start implementing good habits to build a foundation so strong that it overrides your bad habits.

I know, ugh!!! That doesn't sound fun at all! Don't worry—we're going to make it fun. You're going to be your own boss, kick bad habits to the curb, and replace them with good ones. You'll build your mental fortitude—automatically, without all the suffering and sacrifice you've been through a million times before. The goal is a level of happiness and success in your life that you may not have felt before. That's the badass way—and what this book is all about.

This book is a day-by-day motivational guide designed to encourage habit change and mental toughness through fun, dynamic daily tasks. It takes you through a 30-day program with easy-to-implement solutions involving positive daily habits to create a better, well-rounded lifestyle.

It takes 30 days to break a bad habit and 30 days to make a good one. So if you follow my program faithfully, a day at a time, expect to meet a "new badass you" at the end of one month—one amazing phenom who looks great, feels great, and storms the scene with heart and soul.

How badass will you be? Total badass.

My 30-day program shows you how to increase your willpower and self-confidence, overcome negative thinking that has held you back before, and love yourself; it also helps increase your creative and logical thinking. *The Badass Life* will help put the power of your mind, body, and spirit to work for you. This is the whole-package program.

Each day tackles a different subject, with fun activities in different categories that will get you firing on all cylinders. For example:

- Mind work that includes quizzes, life questions, or small challenges that make you think, not just act. These help activate your mind for greater motivation and the ability to overcome obstacles. Your mind is really the "hard drive" of your entire system—the controlling force. The stronger your mind, the stronger your spirit and body will be. I'll emphasize the power of thoughts, for what we think determines the course of our lives, good or bad. When you change your thoughts, you change your world.
- Physical challenges for the day, as well as suggestions for nutritious foods to eat each day to help you understand—and feel—the physical power of healthy eating. Your body is truly your temple—it holds your mind and spirit—and you get only *one*!
- Spirit work for emotional and spiritual wellness. Here I'm talking about your moral compass—your internal GPS that guides you toward doing the right things and connects you to a bigger purpose for your life. It's what gives your life direction and purpose. Your spirit is your spunk.

Here I'll include work on loving and respecting yourself, meditating, journaling what you appreciate about yourself and your life. These practices open your mind to a deeper, better understanding of how to change habits.

Each day you'll work on making a single positive change. One positive change leads to another. Day by day, you work on small behavioral changes like repeating affirmations, learning positive self-talk, setting your day up for success, trying a new type of exercise, and so on. Along the way, you'll notice that you're slowly but surely getting in badass shape—mentally, physically, and spiritually—and feeling phenomenal.

As you go forward, use this book as a workbook, too, writing things down on the pages. Better yet, do it in a personal journal. Once you start journaling, patterns will start to emerge, you'll overcome obstacles to health and fitness, and you'll feel empowered to make positive changes in your life.

Beginner or expert, I have you covered. Just take it one day at a time, and resist the urge to read this book fast or work through each challenge too fast. I outline everything in detail, with lots of tips that will enhance the good habits and loosen the grip of bad habits on your life. You'll work on your mind, body, and spirit every day, and you'll set the stage for what can grow into an amazing badass life. Trust me, stick with it and you'll reach a point when you can't imagine not living like a badass.

After tackling various mental and spiritual challenges, you'll be surprised at how everything in your life starts to fall into place—finances, job challenges, relationships, and more. For years, I've seen the results of all this firsthand: how eating right and working out regularly make you stronger and more vibrant; how being truly honest with yourself and creating accountability systems keep you on track; how goal setting, empowering thoughts, and attitude change seep into other aspects of your life; and how the fitness lifts your spirits and translates into success in everything you do.

So now's the time to ditch the excuses, reach your goals, and even exceed your wildest expectations, using this plan of action and in-the-trenches resolve to turn your dreams into reality. Our mind, bodies, and spirit hold the treasure of life inside of them, life that we have been given. We are good, and we should be treated with honor every day that we are alive. To do that, focus on everything I have for you here. They're simple things, but they're incredibly powerful. If you work at them daily, they can change the precious treasure that is your life. As is true with anything, it just takes some practice, patience, and some belief in this book and yourself.

I feel that we are all on Earth for a purpose and our lives have deep meaning. Discovering that meaning is part of life and motivates us to do all we can to make our lives last as long as possible.

Let the discovery begin!

—*Christmas*

Day 1

BE A POSITIVE GOAL DIGGER— AND AIM *BIG*

*Setting goals is the first step in turning
the invisible into the visible.*
—TONY ROBBINS

SO MANY OF my clients, fans, friends, even family members ask me why they aren't meeting their goals. They claim they're doing everything right to get there . . . whether that means working their asses off in the gym or eating right to lose weight or staying late at the office to earn a promotion. They swear they're doing it all!

For some time, I doubted their claims. I thought to myself: They must be embellishing all their hard work, because there's no way they shouldn't have reached their goals by now. However, after some deep diving into their situations and discussing their goals, I found that there was a significant flaw in their goal-setting process: They were setting *negative goals*.

NEGATIVE GOALS VERSUS POSITIVE GOALS

A negative goal is based on:

- The absence or avoidance of something ("I will cut out bread to lose weight").
- An unrealistic target ("I will start exercising fourteen hours a week").
- A goal that might be harmful ("I will put in eighty-hour workweeks to earn more money").
- Negative reasoning ("If I don't quit smoking, I'll have a stroke").

The act of goal setting itself is crucial to your success. It points you in the direction of your dreams. But if you set goals from a negative point of view, you're setting yourself up for failure. Take weight control, for example, an area where negative goal setting is rampant. One of the reasons weight loss is so tough for a lot of people is that they fixate on everything they can't have; whether it's cake, candy, bread, pasta, desserts, butter, or other foods, they end up craving it, eating it, and blowing the diet. A negative goal might be something like no more refined carbs, no more saturated fats, no more fast food, and so on.

Conversely, a positive goal:

- Focuses on what you will do or have, rather than on what you will not do or what you will avoid. For instance, instead of thinking in terms of avoiding or restricting foods, put your focus on positive goals, such as eating five or more servings of fruits and vegetables a day, eating a quality protein at every meal, or enjoying more energy and a better mood with regular workouts.
- Is realistic. We're all capable of achieving amazing things, but our goals need to be in line with our schedules, skill sets, or genetic makeup. Rather

than saying, "I want to look like Christmas Abbott," make a commitment to weight-train three times a week, 45 minutes per session, or pursue some other physical activity that will eventually create the best physical version of *you.*

- Is attainable. If you make sure your goals can realistically be achieved, you are more likely to reach them. There's no sense in striving to be an NBA player if you're five foot five.

- Has a "when date." This means constructing a realistic deadline for when you will attain your goal or goals. Know what you want to achieve and put a date on it. But be patient. If you're looking to lose body fat and inches, think of how much time it took to put on those pounds or those inches. They will take time to come off.

- Has a known positive outcome. For example, if you want to stop working overtime and getting home late every evening, state your goal like this: "Get home by seven every night to spend more time with my family." Focus on the positive outcome instead of the negative thing that you're trying to avoid, and you'll achieve that goal faster.

- Is framed positively. I once heard someone who was just finishing a boot-camp class say, "This is the best part of the workout—the cooldown!" In contrast, I view my workouts as periods of joy during which I get to play with a bunch of cool toys. Not that I don't take my workouts seriously, but I certainly don't approach them as something to slog through. If the latter describes you, try this: The next time you head toward your gym or get ready to exercise at home, instead of wording your goal as "I have to exercise today," say, "I *get* to exercise today."

THREE TYPES OF DAILY GOALS

As you go through these next 30 days, I'll be asking you to set daily goals and record them in your journal. These should be small, attainable goals that you can work on each day to reach your longer-term larger goals. There are three types of daily goals:

A MENTAL GOAL: Mental goals deal with mental preparation, visualization (see day 5), or productive thinking. Some examples:

I will prepare myself to participate productively in today's meeting.

I have a very clear picture in my mind as to what my body will look like in its optimally developed shape.

I will banish negative thoughts about myself and replace them with positive thoughts.

I will change the way I interpret or respond to stress.

I will practice my daily affirmations.

A PERSONAL GOAL: Personal goals are very concrete and actionable, and have to do with the day-to-day choices you make. For example:

I will eat three servings of vegetables today.

I will work out at the gym for one hour.

I will make it to the finish line.

I will provide a high level of customer service.

I will open a savings account.

A SPIRITUAL GOAL: These focus on personal characteristics to be practiced and developed such as respect, courtesy, loyalty, and friendship. Also, they may include daily spiritual practices that bring you into union with something greater than yourself. Some examples:

I will say my mealtime prayers, do an evening meditation, or read scripture.

I will enjoy a solitary walk.

I will write in my journal.

I will express gratitude to someone in uniform.

I will be a more supportive and dependable friend.

Each day I'll give you examples of these types of goals. You'll have the opportunity to follow those goals, or once you get the hang of daily goal setting, you can create your own.

Goals are like targets, and you have to keep trying to hit them. Imagine your-

MY BADASS REFLECTIONS FOR TODAY

What are you most grateful for today?

Mentally: _____

Physically: _____

Spiritually: _____

What was the biggest success for you today?

Mentally: _____

Physically: _____

Spiritually: _____

What was the biggest challenge for you today? How did you overcome it?

Mentally: _____

Physically: _____

Spiritually: _____

What can you do tomorrow to make it a better day?

Mentally: _____

Physically: _____

Spiritually: _____

CHECKLIST

☐   I completed my habit change exercises.

☐   I made healthy choices today for my mind, body, and spirit.

☐   I've expressed my gratitude for today and all it brings, good and bad.

☐   I've prepared for tomorrow and all the unknowns it might bring.

Day 2
AFFIRM!

I USE A powerful tool that will help you achieve your goals, reinforce a positive attitude, and help you obtain all that you want: affirmations. By definition, affirmations are short, formal statements repeated time and again, either verbally or mentally or in writing, that express your desired condition or outcome. Some examples:

Want to clean up your nutrition and adopt a healthier lifestyle? Tell yourself: "I'm building health and changing my life for me."

Want to quit smoking or drinking? Find momentum with words like "If I can make it a minute, I can make it an hour . . . If I can make it a month, I can make it forever."

Being considered for a new job? You might use something like "I'm going to nail this interview" or "I have the qualifications and the ability to succeed in this position."

Are you thin on finances? Say, "I'm in the process of creating wealth."

Need to move beyond a broken relationship? Repeat the words "I'm an attractive, passionate, loving, and giving person."

Feeling down? Turn it around by repeating an affirmation like "I'm a beautiful person who has a lot to offer the world." Then watch your spirit start to lift.

Affirmations program your mind to line up with your intentions—eat better, exercise more consistently, quit bad habits, get a better job, master your finances, and heal after a relationship ends. Affirmations tap into our subconscious mind and become our beliefs. Your mind believes what you put into it.

But do affirmations truly work? Or are they just a touchy-feely form of mumbo jumbo? Some good news: Psychologists, neuroscientists, and other researchers have discovered in studies that, yes, affirmations really do work.

One study found that when female students in introductory physics classes wrote affirmations to themselves about improving their test performances, their test scores improved dramatically. Another study found that couples who paused at the beginning of an argument to speak affirmations about themselves or aspects of their lives unrelated to the argument were less likely to escalate the fight. Here's another one: British psychologists organized women into two groups. One group was asked to repeat affirmations about eating more fruits and vegetables while the other group (the controls) did not practice any affirmations. Those in the affirmation group ate significantly more portions of fruits and vegetables, leading the researchers to conclude: "Self-affirmation interventions can successfully influence health-promoting behaviors."

Clearly, there's a direct connection. When you tell yourself you're going to succeed at something, those thoughts change your brain to make it happen. In other words, what you think about and speak about will materialize.

How then do you go about developing affirmations?

DECIDE WHAT YOU WANT. Health? Wealth? Loving relationships? A better job?

Be specific. For example, let's say you have an upcoming deadline for an important project. You might say: "I'm going to get this project completed successfully by Monday." Specificity helps us focus our intent and reminds us day to day what we want to be, what is true, and what could be.

WRITE OUT YOUR AFFIRMATIONS. Begin your statements with powerful words. Two of the most powerful words you can use are *I am* because they express your affirmation in the present tense. You want your mind to believe it is happening. For example, "I am healthy because I eat nutritious foods and work out regularly." The next most powerful words are *I can, I will,* and *I have.* For example, if you want a promotion at work, write: "I have everything it takes to be a strong, successful leader."

BE POSITIVE. Speak in terms of what you want instead of what you don't. It's better to say "I am becoming wealthier" than "I don't want to be broke." If you talk about what you don't want, that is exactly what you'll get. You see, we get what we focus on and feel good or bad about, consistently. If you dwell on the stack of bills on your desk and are worried constantly about your budget, for instance, chances are that you'll attract more money problems—which is exactly what you don't want. Why? Because you're not thinking positively and proactively about the situation. Staring at a stack of bills and debts or at your empty wallet sends out negative vibrations, which keep you stuck. So don't dwell on it. Dwell on positives. If you don't like your financial situation, then you and your thoughts have the power to turn it. Tell yourself that you're in the process of building financial security. And while you're at it, connect positive feelings to positive thoughts: *I love the feeling of being debt free.* Be clear about what you want, too—a positive cash flow, a lot of money in the bank, and so forth. The way you think is what you will attract.

TAP INTO OTHERS' WISDOM. If you have trouble creating your own affirmations, look to affirming quotes by others and adapt them. For example:

The more I focus my mind upon the good, the more good comes to me.
—LOUISE HAY

I am creating financial security through the use of my talents.
—MARIANNE MITCHELL

Every circumstance is a chance for you to practice being the
person you truly want to be.
—MARIANNE WILLIAMSON

Believe that life is worth living, and your belief will help create the fact.
—WILLIAM JAMES

I am thankful for all of those who said no to me.
It's because of them I'm doing it myself.
—ALBERT EINSTEIN

We become what we think about.
—EARL NIGHTINGALE

RECITE YOUR AFFIRMATIONS ON A REGULAR BASIS—AT LEAST TWICE A DAY. I suggest you read or say them each morning upon awakening and again each night just before falling asleep—or really any time during the day. I like to post my affirmations in key places, too, in order to remind me what my goal is and how to stay on track. For example:

—Quote on my fridge: "You are beautiful! Stay the course."

—A few favorite quotes on my bathroom mirror: "Today you can make a change," "Prove them wrong!" and "Do today what others won't so you can do tomorrow what others can't."

—Quotes in my car: "Sweat off the fat!" and "I'm doing all this for me!"

BELIEVE YOUR AFFIRMATIONS! Make them a part of you and great things will happen.

If you want to create change in yourself or your life, and develop the mental toughness it takes to succeed at anything, affirmations are a powerful force that you should not underestimate or take for granted. Whatever you want to achieve or change, repeating something as simple as "I can do this" will make you feel like nothing can stand in your way.

For Today

TODAY'S QUOTE

I affirm to you the tremendous potential you have, not beyond anything you could ever imagine.
—STEPHEN COVEY

TODAY'S CHALLENGE

Create your own affirmations. Think about those big fat ridiculous goals you wrote down before, and harness affirmations to support them. Write them down on 3x5-inch cards and keep them with you at all times. Recite and repeat them often. Soon you will believe your new messaging, and you'll be on the way to achieving and becoming all that you desire.

Today's Mental Goal: _____

_____

Today's Personal Goal:_____

_____

Today's Spiritual Goal: _____

_____

MY BADASS REFLECTIONS FOR TODAY

What are you most grateful for today?

Mentally: _____

Physically: _____

Spiritually: _____

What was the biggest success for you today?

Mentally: _____

Physically: _____

Spiritually: _____

What was the biggest challenge for you today? How did you overcome it?

Mentally: _____

Physically: _____

Spiritually: _____

What can you do tomorrow to make it a better day?

Mentally: _____

Physically: _____

Spiritually: _____

CHECKLIST

☐   I completed my habit change exercises.

☐   I made healthy choices today for my mind, body, and spirit.

☐   I've expressed my gratitude for today and all it brings, good and bad.

☐   I've prepared for tomorrow and all the unknowns it might bring.

Day 3

LEARN TO LOVE YOURSELF

"LOVE YOURSELF!" THAT message may sound like something on a bumper sticker, but it's one of the most important pieces of the change-your-life puzzle. Badasses love themselves.

But how do you actually do that? How do you love yourself and appreciate your value in this world? If you struggle with these questions, you've likely been doing so for many years. Feelings of inadequacy often stem from earlier experiences with family, other people, or traumatic events.

I'm an example of this. I came from a crazy background, with amazing parents who were bikers, hippies, and rolling stones. I'm the middle kid of three children, so I am a classic case of feeling ignored. We were brought up in a rebellious background, with a lot of smoking, drinking, and partying. It's not that my parents threw us kids into a raging house party, but we were exposed to a life filled with less than positive choices. Back then, I knew healthier options existed.

I was, however, raised well, with a focus on manners and an awareness of what I should or shouldn't be doing. My parents loved me wholeheartedly, but I was heavily troubled and depressed through my early teens. I made a lengthy series of terrible choices because of it. I started chain-smoking, drinking whenever I could, and playing with drugs of every description, eventually getting my hands on harder drugs, like meth. I kept sabotaging myself with all this madness. I couldn't even claim I was in bad shape, because I didn't know what good shape was. I was destroying my body, my mind, and especially my spirit, and I was barely out of my teens.

In short, I wasn't always as strong-willed, driven, determined, mindful, and creative as I am today, not at all. I was the very opposite. I had no self-esteem. I didn't believe I was worth more than what I was doing. I simply always assumed that I wasn't capable of doing much. I constantly put myself down.

Maybe you're a lot like I was, beating yourself up at every turn and simply not believing you're worthy of anything. Even if we have a success, we find a way to downgrade our efforts, to make them less of an accomplishment in our own eyes. No matter how much I achieved, I'd play it down. This was my life: destructive, dangerous, barely making ends meet, and resigned to what looked like a dark future.

I was on a path to becoming a full-fledged junkie when my mother suggested that I join her in Iraq, where she was employed as a civilian contractor. There was a job opening, and I decided to apply. I had to get clean to pass the drug test, which meant a period of no meth or other hard drugs. It was incredibly difficult, but I passed the test, and luckily, I was hired—initially as a laundry attendant and later moving up to camp operations specialist, doing logistics work. Anyway, off I went to Iraq, during Operation Iraqi Freedom, and was plopped down right in the middle of a desert war zone.

At first it didn't hit me that I was in a war zone. It didn't feel like war. It felt like a work camp, and militant with so many armed soldiers walking around on high alert. Then came *the* mortar attack. Boom, it happened. That's when I realized this was real—really real. Everything at that moment seemed to unfold in slow motion—

what I did, what I didn't do, and exactly what I was thinking. This was the aha moment for me. I walked away from the attack, knowing that I didn't want to die.

I also knew that if I wanted something better—and I did—I needed to make better decisions. But I had no self-worth to do so. Maybe you've had a similar "rocket-attack" revelation but were at a loss, not knowing what to do or where to turn. I'm living proof that you can change.

Over the next three months, I quit smoking and attempted to start hitting the gym. What really hooked me on fitness, however, was an exercise video I watched online. There were these three teeny little women, my size, and they all had beautiful bodies. They were amazing. One girl cried at the end, and I was like, "That's what I want to do! I want to do a workout that makes me want to cry!" Those girls were doing CrossFit.

So I began a CrossFit program right there in Iraq, using the base gym, which was equipped with everything I needed. But change did not come easily. My lungs screamed for oxygen during an attempt to run a mile, compounded by my nasty smoking habit and an aversion to exercise. That mile nearly killed me. I dragged myself back to my quarters, tired and sore. It took me a week to recover. I did not like where I was. But although I was a bunch of broken pieces, I had hope that they could be patched up together again.

I began working out with a group of Special Forces guys who literally wanted to break me. Picture this: little tiny me, at five foot three, so underweight at 95 to 100 pounds that I looked anorexic. You could see the bones in my chest as clearly as on a skeleton. There I was, working out with these big husky macho soldiers! They'd put me through horrific workouts, standing over me to make sure I did every part of the workout and forcing me to finish. What would take them 15 minutes took me 30 to 45 minutes. Barely able to keep up, I was embarrassed to always be the last to finish.

After a few of those grueling workouts, those guys were convinced that I'd stop showing up. But I returned every day, knowing they were waiting for me with a hell workout.

My tenacity and determination to hang in there earned their respect. But really, I learned a valuable lesson from them: *Do not give up, no matter what.* That lesson stuck with me and would become the foundation for success in my life.

What drove me was the thought of going back to my life before the mortar attack. That "before life" terrified me. Had I not decided to change my life, I would have ended up as a junkie. I no longer wanted to invite death into my world. I wanted to crawl out of my rut and see what it was like on the other side. I had no idea what new worlds might await me.

After four years in Iraq, I returned to the United States and began coaching a boot camp and CrossFit classes, eventually opening my own CrossFit gym and competing in CrossFit competitions around the world. Over time, I became convinced that someday I would be part of something bigger than myself and be able to make a difference in the lives of others. I felt propelled along a new course of life.

Maybe you've come to a similar point in your life. If so, you have two options: Stay the course—aka, do nothing—or make some major changes in your life. If you choose the latter, know this: Small steps lead to miles walked and great heights. It took me more than a decade to climb my own mountain, and I didn't start at the base of the mountain, either. I started in the ditches, below ground level, almost buried under a burden of a decade of poor decisions and feelings of worthlessness. Nor was this life change perfect from day 1. I relapsed a lot and struggled with insecurities. It was slow progress, with one step forward and one step back. Sometimes it was two steps forward, two steps back. But at least I was pushing myself forward.

If you're truly ready to change, as I was, it does involve learning to love yourself. So, back to the original question: How do you do that? How do you move forward and create self-love?

I have a simple secret: Lie to yourself! This is also known as "faking the funk." That's what I did from the get-go. I simply lied. I call this *find your lioness*, otherwise called your *lying-ness*.

This isn't lying in the way you think it is. It isn't being untrue to yourself or inauthentic in the way you live. Rather, it is lying to those voices in your head that are telling you that you aren't worth it, that you're not as good as other people, that you're a failure, that you're not smart enough, and all that BS.

Negative statements like these can be devastating to your self-confidence and stand in the way of your loving yourself. The problem is that your subconscious mind begins to believe that you're worthless and unlovable, and it makes you act as if those messages are really true. Negative thinking develops into a habit—one that gets so deeply entrenched in your psyche that you're not even aware of it. And it cheats you out of happiness and success!

Naturally, you feel like retreating. You may pick up a glass of wine, a bottle of bourbon, a pack of smokes, a whole cake, or some other temporary "thrill" in an attempt to silence the whir of negativity. But these things don't offer real reprieve; they only contribute to and compound the mess in your mind.

There are easier ways to break these negative habits and make positive new habits of self-love and self-confidence. Just as your subconscious mind believes the rotten stuff you tell it about yourself, it also believes the wonderful things you say to it. Start doing that now! Here's how to "lie" to yourself:

Ditch your self-bashing mindset. Begin by countering every negative thought about yourself the instant it comes up. If you catch yourself saying:

"I'm a failure!"
"I can't!"
"I'm afraid of _____."

Cancel those thoughts and instead say:
"Keep going for one more _____."
"I am a capable person!"
"This is why I'm here!"
"I'm confident I can _____."

Statements like these may feel a little silly or a waste of time, but soon you'll believe them, and soon after that, they'll become true. Then watch how quickly your feelings about yourself and the situation begin to change. If you start altering your thoughts, you start changing your attitude, and you ultimately change the way you see yourself and the way you act.

Believe it or not, I used to feel very insecure and self-conscious about my body—even after I built some serious muscle and curves! I'd walk into a restaurant in a strapless minidress with my chiseled arms and legs bare for all to see. The whole time I'd be worried about what people were thinking (*she's got too much muscle, she's too bulky*, and so on). I finally had to banish these crazy approval-seeking thoughts from my mind and replace them with thoughts like *I feel proud that my hard work has warranted some attention*, and I smile at the onlookers. As a result, the coolest stuff happens. People now approach me with compliments, and they ask me about my fitness regimen and diet—which I am always happy to talk about.

So start cranking up your own ego. It may sound cheesy, but keep a running list in your head of all the reasons why you're a badass—you can blast out squat reps like nobody's business, your opinion is highly respected in business meetings, you can glam up with the best of them, everyone wants to dance with you because you're so damn good, your Tinder matches are piling up, and they all want dates. Repeating the list to yourself can ratchet up your confidence and self-love, anytime, anyplace.

Fake it until you make it. Lie to yourself by "acting as if" you have certain qualities that you may not yet have. Act as if you're that happy, self-confident, independent person, that you're worth the workout, worth the effort to get fit, worth so much more than you have given yourself credit for. Be like those actors who get so caught up in their roles that they practically become the characters they portray. Well, taking on a confident, badass persona can help you feel superconfident and in control. If you make a conscious effort to act that way, eventually you'll begin to believe it. Before long, you're not just acting it, you *are* it.

Also, acting happy and confident creates a brain chemistry in which feel-good chemicals called endorphins increase, along with immune-building T cells. Scientists can even do scans of the brain, measure these chemicals, and actually see what anger, sadness, and even happiness look like. So act happy. Laugh. Smile. All these actions activate positive chemicals in your brain that keep you alert, upbeat, and physically healthy.

Loving yourself is the key to almost every success—it can bring you the body you want, the partner of your dreams, the job of your choice, and a circle of wonderful friends. Find your lioness, learn to love yourself, and see your life change fast.

For Today

TODAY'S QUOTE

When I was around eight, I looked in the mirror and said, "You're either going to love yourself or hate yourself." And I decided to love myself. That changed a lot of things.
—QUEEN LATIFAH

TODAY'S AFFIRMATION

_____

_____

_____

TODAY'S CHALLENGE

Practice thought-stopping. This is an action-oriented technique to get rid of those nagging thoughts that haunt us and break unhealthy patterns or habits. Here's what to do:

- Become aware of the messages that stream through your mind and recognize that you're having a negative, unloving thought.
- Wear a rubber band on your wrist and snap it whenever the negative thoughts enter. This is important because it disrupts the negativity and prevents it from growing stronger. By doing this, you shift your mind away from the negative thoughts.

- Shift your mind to a loving thought about yourself. Exchange negative inner dialogue with positive, self-loving statements. Example: "I can't do anything right" versus "I do most things exceptionally well."

Today's Mental Goal:

_____

Today's Personal Goal:

_____

Today's Spiritual Goal:

_____

MY BADASS REFLECTIONS FOR TODAY

What are you most grateful for today?

Mentally: _____

Physically: _____

Spiritually: _____

What was the biggest success for you today?

Mentally: _____

Physically: _____

Spiritually: _____

What was the biggest challenge for you today? How did you overcome it?

Mentally: _____

Physically: _____

Spiritually: _____

What can you do tomorrow to make it a better day?

Mentally: _____

Physically: _____

Spiritually: _____

CHECKLIST

☐   I completed my habit change challenges.

☐   I made healthy choices today for my mind, body, and spirit.

☐   I've expressed my gratitude for today and all it brings, good and bad.

☐   I've prepared for tomorrow and all the unknowns it might bring.

Day 4

EXERCISE YOUR MIND AND SPIRIT

HABITS ARE STUBBORN. It's tough to make an old habit disappear. Once it's wired into your brain, it's stuck there for a long time. But you can override it. You can come up with new, healthier behaviors and weaken the power of old, counterproductive habits on your life.

One of the most effective behaviors for busting bad habits is exercise. People who make exercise a habit start eating better. They also stop using their credit cards quite so much. They stop procrastinating so much at work. There's something life-changing about exercise that echoes throughout our minds and spirit.

In 2014, a group of Chinese researchers analyzed twenty-two studies to determine how effective long-term exercise could be as a treatment for substance abuse disorders, including pain pill addiction, alcohol abuse, smoking, and use of illicit hard drugs such as cocaine and heroin. The results of the analysis were incredibly hopeful and encouraging. Addicts who exercised regularly—either through aerobic activity or mind-body work like yoga, tai chi, or qigong—abstained from their addictions, were less depressed and anxious, and had fewer withdrawal symptoms.

Drug dependency is a habit that at its worst is superdifficult to kick. If exercise can help kick the most terrible habits of all, as this study shows, imagine what it can do to wipe out other less serious but frustrating habits that are holding you back?

You know how you feel after a really great workout—strong and renewed and bursting with energy? Well, in addition to keeping your body strong and flexible, exercise does wonders for your mind and spirit. It boosts self-esteem, gives you the satisfaction of striving for and attaining your goals, and helps keep the blues at bay. There are hundreds of studies that prove all of this.

Why is exercise so powerful for mental health? Exercise actually functions like a drug. It increases the release of mood-boosting endorphins in the brain and it boosts levels of other feel-good brain chemicals, such as serotonin and dopamine. Both are involved in regulating moods, in enhancing brain skills like thinking and memory, and in producing sensations of pleasure.

Exercise is a natural stress reliever, too. If you're angry, peeved, or frustrated, rather than fuming at someone or reaching for a few drinks, release that stress with a workout. A half hour on a bike or treadmill, circuit training on weight machines, pounding a punching bag, or working out to a fitness video or a YouTube channel will help you let off steam.

Exercise is great for the spirit, too. Sure, the changes in your physique are exciting, but you'll begin to notice that not only do you feel better physically but you feel better spiritually as well. You'll have more spiritual energy—the feeling that what you do in life matters. Practices like yoga can even leave you with a spiritual high.

WHAT YOU CAN DO

To harness the benefits of this natural habit breaker, antidepressant, stress buster, and spiritual booster, I support several types of exercise.

FOCUS ON AEROBIC FITNESS. It doesn't matter how strong you are or how good your jump shot is if you can't breathe. You're working out aerobically when your breathing accelerates, your blood flows faster, and your heart pumps more of it, sending nutrients and oxygen to the rest of your body. Get in at least three aerobic workouts a week (stair climbing, walking, treadmill work, running, and so forth) and you'll see your mood and anxiety levels improve. Try to increase your time, distance, and speed each week. Here are some of my favorite badass cardio suggestions:

HOOF IT UP A HILL. Find a hilly area in your community and do some walking or running up those hills. Push off your heels as you go. Enjoy the outdoors; it can be a spiritual encounter with nature.

DO SOME CYCLING. Increase the resistance to high on a stationary bike and sit toward the back of your seat to fully engage your hamstrings and glutes. Try a recumbent bike or regular cycling; both are great workouts.

CLIMB STAIRS. Find a local stadium where you can go up and down the bleachers, or try a stair climber at the gym. Climb at a challenging incline and try not to put too much of your weight on the handrails. Leaning too heavily on the rails deprives you of a good cardiovascular workout and risks injury to your hands and wrists.

GO CROSS-COUNTRY SKIING. It's absolutely the best cardio and toning outdoor workout for your entire body. Outdoor workouts are among the most exhilarating ways to get a spiritual high because you're in close contact with nature. Or work out on a cross-country ski machine for a mental and spiritual lift.

GET IN THE POOL. Use a kickboard and do as many laps as you can of flutter and butterfly kicks. There's something soothing about being in the water.

BUILD MUSCLE, BUILD SELF-ESTEEM. You gotta get strong, but it's not just to build your body; it's also to build your self-esteem and body image. In an experiment with female volunteers, a Brigham Young University study found that weight training significantly improved self-esteem and body image, compared to a non-weight-training control group. This was in part due to significant improvements in body composition and lean muscle. Women like how they looked, and they felt more self-confident and self-loving because their bodies had changed for the better. I see the same results at my gym all the time: When people get stronger through lifting weights, they experience a level of self-confidence greater than that of people who don't lift.

A really great example of what I'm talking about is one of my gym members, Alicia. After hitting her early forties, she watched her body gradually change, with fat creeping on her booty and belly. Plus, she was experiencing a lot of fatigue. She no longer felt sexy and was desperate for a change.

Alicia had always done mostly cardio classes—so I immediately plunged her into weight training, and I mean with barbells, mostly, and multi-muscle moves such as squats and deadlifts (great for tightening the booty). She was a little hesitant at first, but admitted she wanted strong, sexy muscles. So I said, "Fine, if that's what you want, you've got to train with heavy weights—and eat right to create that kind of muscle."

Alicia turned out to be such a great student. She not only achieved the badass body she wanted but also developed a badass persona and an obvious mental toughness. She was more self-assured and thoroughly committed to the badass lifestyle. As she told me: "I am confident. I have the energy to power through my workouts and days, and I've never felt stronger and sexier in my life! I love my new badass self!!!"

So definitely include weights or strength-building exercises into your routine. To make progress, physically and mentally, you have to fight hard for every new ounce of muscle. This is what I had to do. Before becoming a badass in competitions, I focused on the fundamentals of lifting and setting up my life in a very organized fashion so that I could master them.

A lot of people skip this step; they want to fast-track through the "boring" fundamentals. Not me! I knew that pushing my body would require mastery of the simplest moves before moving on to more complicated ones. By becoming so good at the core foundation movements, I was able to learn and excel at the more advanced levels of lifting and competing.

I compare this process to building your dream home. There are many details that come with that: cabinet colors, tile styles, window frames, molding, and so forth. But none of that matters unless you first build the proper foundation, the proper reinforcements, and a strong frame. Then and only then can you add the bells and whistles of decor. Likewise, you simply can't build a strong regimen by rushing through the basic foundations of training.

By the time I started to compete, my movements were stronger, my muscular endurance was faster, and I was surpassing women and men who were actually stronger and faster than I was. By sticking with and learning the fundamentals, I pushed my limits in speed and strength while maintaining good, safe form.

Once you've mastered the basics, continually challenge yourself to do more, but without substantially increasing the time you spend training. For a muscle to grow, the training stimulus must be progressively increased. That may mean more weight, reps, or sets. This is the other way I fight hard for muscles and strength.

And stay focused on the act of working out itself. No mind wandering! By simply thinking about your action as you do it, you increase its quality tenfold.

Constantly change up your workouts, too. If you've been doing the same old exercises, sets, and reps week in and week out, your muscles may stop responding. Try some new exercises, or new sequences of performing them, or any other method you can think of to mix it up. The more your body is forced to overcome a new stimulus, the more you create muscle tone, growth, strength— and greater self-confidence.

EASE ANXIETY WITH PLYOMETRICS. Plyometrics (jumping exercises) are helpful when you need a sudden burst of speed or in sports, like basketball, that require quick directional change. My favorite plyometrics exercise is jumping rope, the way you did as a kid. Remember all those crazy tricks—monkey in the middle, double Dutch, hopscotch? Why not try them again?

Some tips: Relax your shoulders as you jump. Keep your elbows pinned by your sides to ensure the rope remains the same length and same distance above your head and under your feet at all times. Stay light on your toes—gently bounce up and down. Don't let your feet sink into the floor, and jump in one spot straight up and down. And don't forget to breathe! Inhale and exhale at a steady rate throughout the movement.

I don't know of any research that shows that plyometrics give you a mental boost, but I do know that it's a playful activity that brings out the kid in me—and that relieves anxiety and worry immediately.

Other plyometric exercises include jumping squats, jumping lunges, explosive push-ups, clapping push-ups, and burpees. Instructions for performing these can be found in my book *The Badass Body Diet*.

MIND-BODY WORK. Yoga is my favorite; plus, it's a proven habit breaker. It helps free patients from addictions because it stimulates relaxation, eases muscle tension, and fosters positive mental and spiritual health.

A Swedish study published in 2014 in *Complementary Therapies in Medicine* explored whether yoga could work as part of a treatment program for alcohol-dependent patients. For ten weeks, patients took part in weekly group yoga session and were encouraged to practice yoga at home once a day. The members of a control group did not do yoga. Both groups underwent traditional therapy. By the end of the study, the yoga group cut back their daily drinking from six to three drinks daily, while the control group continued to drink heavily. The researchers concluded that yoga was definitely effective in helping people ease off alcohol.

Similar evidence has been found in smokers. University of Cincinnati researchers analyzed a bunch of studies involving yoga and smoking cessation. Most of the studies showed that yoga helped smokers quit. Their analysis was published in the *Journal of Evidence-Based Complementary & Alternative Medicine* in 2014.

Yoga rocks! So grab a yoga mat and go. Who knows? After a few classes, you might even get addicted to yoga and rid yourself of nasty habits. If you're new to yoga, most gyms and fitness centers offer beginner yoga, gentle yoga, or basic yoga classes. Another type of easy-to-learn yoga is yin yoga, which focuses on a lot of light stretching poses held for longer periods of time.

CROSS-TRAIN. This means incorporating all of the above—aerobics, strength training, plyometrics, and some mind-body exercise—into your workouts. Cross-Fit is designed around this principle, encouraging exercisers to bounce between lifting, hauling, sprinting, jumping, climbing, and practically anything else the human body can do—and that's why I love it so much.

MAKE IT FUN. When I prepare for competition, I have the best excuse to be in the gym all day, every day. Still, it has to be fun for me. There's a saying: "If the love of what you do exceeds the effort of doing it, success is inevitable." Whatever the activity, make sure it's fun.

For Today

TODAY'S QUOTE

I do have to take care of myself, not only because I'm in the movies, just for mental health reasons. I exercise for me. You know, maybe it would be nice to not have to do that in order to feel good, but I do. I feel like I have to, to feel good.
—ANNETTE BENING

TODAY'S AFFIRMATION

_____

_____

_____

TODAY'S CHALLENGE

Sometimes you've just got to tune out the garbage and focus on you and your goals. A perfect way to do this is to take a "walking meditation" today. A walking meditation can be as effective as a sitting meditation, and helps bring strong awareness to your body and mind. Here's how:

- Choose a path on which to walk, preferably a safe area that brings you in contact with nature—the beach, the woods, or a special outdoor walking path.
- As you walk, consciously bring your attention to your body. Notice the sensations of your feet on the ground, the sun and breeze on your skin, the color of the leaves and flowers around you.
- Focus on your goals—how important it is for you to become fit, healthy, and energized.
- Repeat to yourself a prayer, an affirmation, a chant, or a simple word or phrase that you find sacred, like *peace*, *shalom*, *love*, or *om*, or a poem you've memorized that has deep meaning for you.
- If you begin to think of something distracting, bring your focus back to your mind, body, and spirit.

Today's Mental Goal:

_____

Today's Personal Goal:

_____

Today's Spiritual Goal:

_____

MY BADASS REFLECTIONS FOR TODAY

What are you most grateful for today?

Mentally: _____

Physically: _____

Spiritually: _____

What was the biggest success for you today?

Mentally: _____

Physically: _____

Spiritually: _____

What was the biggest challenge for you today? How did you overcome it?

Mentally: _____

Physically: _____

Spiritually: _____

What can you do tomorrow to make it a better day?

Mentally: _____

Physically: _____

Spiritually: _____

CHECKLIST

☐   I completed my habit change challenges.

☐   I made healthy choices today for my mind, body, and spirit.

☐   I've expressed my gratitude for today and all it brings, good and bad.

☐   I've prepared for tomorrow and all the unknowns it might bring.

Day 5
VISUALIZE!

I BELIEVE IN visualization, a relatively old concept in the field of sport psychology. It's been widely used by athletes and others to actualize their potential and improve performance. A golfer, for instance, might visualize a perfect swing, or an actor might visualize an Oscar-winning performance.

In fact, I use visualization all the time when I'm preparing to compete in CrossFit events, particularly in Olympic Weightlifting, where I compete at the 53-kilo level. For background, it involves performing movements called the snatch and the clean and jerk. With the snatch, you hoist a barbell off the floor in one continuous motion over your head. Next you pull your whole body under it so that you're squatting with your elbows locked in extension with the weight overhead; then you stand to finish the lift.

The clean and jerk are two movements performed in one session. With the clean, you pull the weighted barbell to your shoulders. Immediately afterward you do the jerk, by hoisting the same weight overhead and finishing in a standing position with the weight overhead.

Prior to a competition, I picture myself performing these moves with perfect form and superhuman strength. It's all I think about, and I make it vivid and sensory. I visualize everything—the smell of the contest floor, the taste of the sweat as it drips into my mouth, the sounds of my breathing as I lift. I go through every single detail of the lifts so many times that often I feel physically exhausted! By the time I step up there to actually lift the weight, it feels as if I've already done it—and I've won.

Remember what I explained earlier: If you do something repeatedly, the brain secretes chemicals that cause dendrites on the brain cells related to the action to grow until they connect with one another, forming in a new network. When this growth is complete, the brain has the most efficient possible wiring to enable the action. What psychologists have discovered is that simply imagining the activity (visualization) has almost the same effect. The mind doesn't seem to care if you are physically performing the action or simply imagining it.

Visualization is very powerful. You can use it to break bad habits, form new ones, and get the results you want. Here are some examples of how to harness its power.

IN YOUR PROFESSIONAL LIFE

Success in business or on your job has to do with what you create in your mind. Industrialist Henry Ford once hired an efficiency expert to evaluate the running of his company. The expert's report was favorable, although he expressed concern about one employee. "It's that man down the corridor," he said. "Every time I go by his office, he's just sitting there with his feet on his desk. He's wasting your money."

"That man," replied Ford, "once had an idea that saved us millions of dollars. At the time, I believe his feet were planted right where they are now."

That Ford employee was visualizing—a form of creative daydreaming still used today by many corporations to create new products, find solutions to tough prob-lems, and address other business challenges.

With visualization, you go inside your mind to mentally rehearse the perfect outcome of a situation—say, a sales call or a presentation you must make—before you actually do it. You imagine yourself answering any and all questions that the prospect may ask, so that when these questions arise, you are prepared, and you see yourself doing it confidently and articulately. The same goes for giving the presen-tation. You mentally rehearse everything in your mind—your posture, your words, the confidence you display, the way you move from point to point without a hitch. If you visualize often and well enough, when you actually make the call or give the speech, you'll pull it off brilliantly because you've practiced it in your mind.

IN FITNESS

Working toward your ideal body? Find a quiet environment without any distrac-tions and take a comfortable seated position. Close your eyes and relax your mus-cles. Begin to think about your physique. Visualize each problem area you'd like to improve—abs, butt, thighs, and so forth—and form a picture in your mind's eye of the way you want them to look. See yourself walking on the beach in a bikini, strutting around in tight skinny jeans and heels, or wearing a sexy dress to a party. Make the image as clear and realistic as possible.

Here's the thing: Your subconscious mind wants to prove you right. Tell it that you are slim and that you can maintain your ideal weight, and that will become your reality. The more you visualize a buff, fit you, the more your mind works to create it. What the mind believes, you can achieve.

You can also visualize intense, productive workouts. See yourself in your mind's eye dominating those weights with unrestricted strength, forcing out that last rep or two, flexing like a pretzel in yoga class, or running along a route with the fresh air on your skin. Concentrate on these images.

This mental imagery can help your mind focus on your upcoming workout. You'll find, too, that it will improve your intensity, muscle growth, and mind power. You're more likely to increase the weights you lift, the number of sets you perform, or your duration on the treadmill.

Another visualization technique: As you slip into your workout clothes, visualize that you're also symbolically changing into your "workout identity." Imagine that you're changing into a more powerful alter ego, like Diana Prince morphing into Wonder Woman, or Clark Kent changing into Superman. You're not the person who sits at home or at a desk all day; you're the superhero who can wield amazing powers when necessary!

Not only will these exercise-focused visualizations help you boost your fitness, they will also silence the loud internal voice we hear once in a while that says, "Turn the car in the direction of that fast-food joint"—and form new pathways in the brain that keep you motivated and on course.

FOR YOUR SPIRITUAL LIFE

From a spiritual perspective, visualization can be a way to find inner peace. Imagine yourself lying on a breeze-caressed tropical beach, picnicking at the base of a snowcapped mountain, or walking through a tree-canopied forest. You can visualize all sorts of imaginary venues where there is sanctuary from the stresses of modern life.

Another form of spiritual visualization is prayer and meditation. Making time to be with God, Spirit, or a higher power in the rush of pressures that claim your attention—that's what delivers you from those pressures, and why spiritual visualization can be so powerful.

What do you want in your life? Spiritual visualization also borrows from the biblical teaching of "ask, believe, and receive." In your mind, create the picture of what you want, feel it, and hold it intently in your mind. Ask for it. Believe you will receive it. See yourself receiving it. Your thoughts, combined with your feelings and requests, create a sort of "magnet." This magnet attracts experiences that match your thoughts and feelings. If you desire something really strongly and keep your focus on it, you will most likely obtain it.

The mind has considerable influence over the rest of the body, which is why visualization has been applied in many endeavors—to increase people's public speaking ability, to help them quit smoking or drinking, even to shrink tumors. The possibilities are unlimited because visualizations come from your imagination. With visualization, you can develop a subconscious confidence in your abilities that can improve your actions in the real task. That's because your subconscious cannot tell fantasy from reality. Everything you need is right inside you—as long as you believe in yourself and see yourself achieving your goals and dreams.

For Today

TODAY'S QUOTE

Visualization—it's been huge for me. Your mind doesn't know the difference between imagination and reality. You can't always practice perfectly—my fingers will play a little bit out of tune, or my dance moves might not be as sharp—but in my mind, I can practice perfectly.
—LINDSEY STIRLING

TODAY'S AFFIRMATION

_____

_____

_____

Pick a visualization. Go over what we talked about today. Select something you'd like to visualize: a productive workout, a better body, or another goal you'd like to achieve. Find your preferred environment. Some people can visualize anywhere—in a crowded room, on a train, in the line at the grocery store; others prefer a quiet setting. Then simply create an image in your mind of your achieving that goal. Revisit that image frequently throughout the day, especially at night before you go to sleep.

Immerse yourself in sensory details. You can make your visualization come true if you attach emotion and feeling to it. For example, if you are about to do a triathlon; recall the first time you jumped on a bike as a kid and how thrilling it was! You felt the wind in your hair, the excitement of keeping your balance, and the pride of your accomplishment. Transfer that excitement into visualizing success at the triathlon. Think about how it feels to perform at your peak. Your heart rate picks up. Your body is in motion. You're sweating. And you've moving in sync with the sport. Visualize all the details of your performance, with the best possible outcome. Imagine finishing the race, crossing the finish line, taking your prize, sharing hugs with your family and teammates, and basking in the glory of all your hard work paying off. When we visualize and add feeling, we create a possibility of achievement.

Try guided visualizations, too. To help you practice visualization, to add something new to this exercise, or to just take it up a notch, get your hands on a guided imagery program. Guided imagery is a program of directed thoughts and suggestions in which you are led by an instructor in person or on a CD or online. Guided imagery has been used to help people break addictions, eat healthier, and relieve stress and anxiety, among other issues. Many community health centers offer guided imagery classes, or you can search online for CDs or videos.

Today's Mental Goal:

_____

Today's Personal Goal:

_____

Today's Spiritual Goal:

_____

MY BADASS REFLECTIONS FOR TODAY

What are you most grateful for today?

Mentally: _____

Physically: _____

Spiritually: _____

What was the biggest success for you today?

Mentally: _____

Physically: _____

Spiritually: _____

What was the biggest challenge for you today? How did you overcome it?

Mentally: _____

Physically: _____

Spiritually: _____

What can you do tomorrow to make it a better day?

Mentally: _____

Physically: _____

Spiritually: _____

CHECKLIST

☐   I completed my habit change challenges.

☐   I made healthy choices today for my mind, body, and spirit.

☐   I've expressed my gratitude for today and all it brings, good and bad.

☐   I've prepared for tomorrow and all the unknowns it might bring.

Day 6
PREPARE TO SUCCEED—DAILY

MY LIFE INVOLVES a lot of interaction with people. I train clients at my Cross-Fit gym, I run a business in which I represent athletes, I give nutrition and training seminars all over the world, and I compete in regional and national CrossFit events. Wherever I go, I love meeting people and getting to know them, and I'm often asked, "How do you do everything you do?"

It makes me chuckle, because, well, I wonder the same thing. That's because my mind is often chaotic, with thoughts bouncing around like a bunch of tennis balls in a dryer. Yet I stay focused, organized, and turbocharged.

That's because I *structure* my days. I think about *how* I will succeed, not *if.* We humans thrive on structure, even the chaotic ones like me! I may not initially *want* to do something, but when I have a system in place, even the smallest one, things get on track and they get done right. So most of my life consists of regular routines and steady disciplines—my daily rituals. These lead to success in daily living.

One of the most important of those rituals is that I prepare the night before. If it's going to be successful, tomorrow has to start tonight. Before I go to bed, I do two things. First, I reflect on my day. You'll never make the most of the day that's coming until you evaluate the day that has passed. Who did I help? What did I accomplish? What did I learn? Did I do my best?

Second, I look at the next day to see what I need to get done—within the daily agenda I live by. Is there something I should prioritize tomorrow? What will be the main event? What really matters tomorrow? Then I commit to giving my all to that important thing or things. I don't try to prioritize my whole life; I just prioritize my day.

As for that day, my schedule doesn't vary too much, unless I'm traveling. I'll walk you through my typical day and teach you how to make yours as effective as possible. It looks something like this:

5:00 A.M.: Wake up, walk my bulldog, Fran, and have breakfast. (On weekends, I have a different schedule.) After breakfast, I put on my workout clothes and get ready to head to the gym.

6:00 A.M.: Work out.

7:30 A.M.: Shower, stretch, meditate. Two or three times a week, I'll do yoga or ROMWOD (a workout that improves my range of motion).

8:30–11:00 A.M.: Write and create nutritional and workout programs for my clients and my website. No emails!

11:00 A.M–12:30 P.M./1:00 P.M.: Eat lunch, then do my meal prep for dinner. (This involves segmenting out the protein, carbohydrates, and fats I'll have for my evening meal. Getting this done at lunch saves me tons of time at night.)

1:00–5:00 P.M.: Take care of business, including answering emails, reviewing contracts, handling social media and other promotions, checking financials, meetings, updating projects. The rest of the day varies. Sometimes I'll be doing nutrition seminars. Other times I'll be training clients or leading exercise classes. Or I'll write. Or I'll be brainstorming future projects and mapping them out.

5:00–7:00 P.M.: Run errands, cook dinner, or spend playtime with Fran.

7:00–9:00 P.M.: Eat dinner and enjoy family time.

9:00 P.M.: Bedtime.

No matter what your personal daily schedule, I believe that it's key to create a list of tasks in order of priority so as to get things accomplished efficiently. What I like to do is to put my list into three categories. *Hot* tasks are the first group. These tasks are urgent, have to be completed by a deadline (such as bills, book deadlines, booking travel for an event, my workouts, and so forth) and are critical to my life and business. I've got to attend to them quickly, and I get them done first.

Second is my *warm* list. These are important tasks, but may have deadlines that are further out. Important tasks are those that, once completed, help me achieve my daily or monthly goals. Examples include running errands or planning meal schedules.

Finally, I have my *cold* list. These are tasks I'd like to get done. There's no deadline attached to them, and I can push them back if I need to (such as cleaning up files or reorganizing spaces). Sometimes I can delegate these activities to another person.

Once you take the time to create a priority task list, you'll get the most important things done in a timely manner. This translates into better performance, less stress, and more success in all areas of your life.

Schedules and priority task lists really work! Because I wake up knowing how I will spend my day, I can hit the ground running. I've prepared myself to succeed—that day. Whatever the day holds, I try to give my best and be as effective in the moment as I can.

The consequences of living like this are amazing. For example, I discovered that if I work out at six A.M., before the chaos of the day, I'm more mindful as I go through the rest of my day. I was *not* a six A.M. person to start with. Getting up this early took commitment—and going to bed much earlier, of course. That was hard, since I was normally a night owl, but I knew that it would help enhance my day and create a better, more balanced schedule. Eventually it became a part of my daily routine and a positive new habit. Now I love my six A.M. workouts.

I'm not suggesting that if you're a night owl you need to change your schedule as radically as I did, nor that you necessarily do early-morning workouts. Hey, a lot of people aren't early risers or morning folks. I get that. You've really got to figure out a schedule that works for your lifestyle. Two things to consider: Work your schedule so that you get at least seven to eight hours of sleep, so that your body will be properly restored. Then listen to your body: Are you stronger when you do afternoon or evening workouts, and less energetic or focused during workouts at other times? Do your exercising at the times your body responds the best.

Also, think about the series of events in your day and what you normally do. Do you wake up to the alarm at a certain time, hit the snooze button once or twice, and then go back to sleep, only to become increasingly later for the rest of the day? Or do you spring out of bed? Do you eat before you shower and brush your teeth or the other way around? Have you set out your clothes for the day, packed your gym bag in advance, and prepped healthy meals and snacks? Do you have a schedule for your routines and daily activities or do you just wing all of them? Your daily routine reflects your habits, good or bad.

Prepare for success consistently every day and your old bad habits will lose their grip over you. Through discipline and practice of the new habit, the old habit fades out of view. It might want to reappear, but it is relegated to the background. Your new habits become second nature, and the idea of not acting on them is so remote that you forget you ever had bad habits.

With a little bit of awareness, you can create better habits and ultimately better preparation for the day and life ahead. All it takes is a little *front-end effort*. Here are some things to think about as you plan your day.

- Thoughts: Practice self-loving thoughts throughout the day. My personal self-loving mantra is "I'm the baddest bitch here!" This might sound a little intrusive, maybe even cocky, but it's played a huge factor in my success.
- Life management: Properly manage your work, finances, goals, household, and schedule. Decide, for example, when you will answer emails. Create your priority task list for the day that covers these aspects of life management. A detailed list with realistic time slots for each task sets you up for huge success on your daily planning. Be sure to include extra time for your habit homework and add in "buffer" time for any unforeseen circumstances like heavy traffic or a mini disaster. I realize this advice might be tough if you've got kids or an on-call type of job. You're going to have to be a little more flexible with your time slots. My recommendation is to figure out when you're most likely to have distraction-free blocks of time and focus on your priorities during those times. You might have to set a realistic limit on the number of outside activities your kids are involved in, too. And if workout time is a problem, get a family gym membership so you can go to the gym together. Your kids can play a sport while you're working out on the gym floor. Above all, be realistic about what you can and cannot accomplish in a day.
- Spirituality: Take time to nurture your faith, spend time in nature, or meditate. Do acts of good without expecting a return, especially when you don't feel like it.
- Nutrition: Fix your meals with the emphasis on clean foods—good proteins, carbs, and fats. You can prep your lunch for the next day right after you finish dinner. Decide, too, when you will eat meals and snacks.
- Exercise: Figure out when is the best time for physical activity and schedule it in. Physical activity could mean playing a sport, working out, or having active fun.
- Health: Invest in self-care daily. This involves dental care, skin care, and quality sleep (including when you will go to bed and when you will wake up). And don't forget your annual physical and routine dental appointments. If you've slacked off on those, pick up the phone today and get them scheduled.

Your life doesn't have to be a minute-to-minute account of what you need to do, but you do need to schedule time at least for meals, exercise, work, and life management priorities, and time for family, fun, and reflection on what matters.

And don't forget: When you reach the end of your day, think about it. Have you lived that day in a healthy, positive way? Have you have done something to improve your life? Have you enriched the lives of others? Your day doesn't have to be perfect; a good day is still a *good day!* Mission accomplished.

For Today

TODAY'S QUOTE

The best preparation for tomorrow is doing your best today.
—H. JACKSON BROWN, JR.

TODAY'S AFFIRMATION

_____

_____

_____

TODAY'S CHALLENGE

Make a plan for today. List your priorities in terms of hot, warm, and cold. Every time you complete one of your priority tasks, check it off and congratulate yourself. Get in the practice of making these lists each day.

Today's Mental Goal:

_____

Today's Personal Goal:

_____

Today's Spiritual Goal:

_____

MY BADASS REFLECTIONS FOR TODAY

What are you most grateful for today?

Mentally: _____

Physically: _____

Spiritually: _____

What was the biggest success for you today?

Mentally: _____

Physically: _____

Spiritually: _____

What was the biggest challenge for you today? How did you overcome it?

Mentally: _____

Physically: _____

Spiritually: _____

What can you do tomorrow to make it a better day?

Mentally: _____

Physically: _____

Spiritually: _____

CHECKLIST

- ☐ I completed my habit change challenges.

- ☐ I made healthy choices today for my mind, body, and spirit.

- ☐ I've expressed my gratitude for today and all it brings, good and bad.

- ☐ I've prepared for tomorrow and all the unknowns it might bring.

Day 7

BE A
RELENTLESS
REBEL

WHERE WOULD WE be if we listened to all the people who tell us what we can't do or what we can't dream? They've been talking to me for years, beginning with a grade school teacher who constantly told me I was an underachiever. For a long time I listened to people like her, but finally their "advice" fell on deaf ears. I no longer make room in my life for naysayers and pessimists. I'm proud to say that my success in CrossFit, NASCAR, business, and elsewhere stems from the fact that I'm a relentless rebel at heart—unwilling to let others decide who I am and what I stand for and willing to pave my own way in this world.

I use the term *relentless rebel* a lot; it's one of my favorite phrases and one that I think describes me best. So what exactly does it mean to be relentless, much less a relentless rebel? It means that you refuse to listen to negative people or see things or events as failures.

Relentless rebels are like my dog, Fran, with a bone in her mouth. The more I try to take away the bone, the harder she clamps down. When we don't get the results we seek, we are simply more motivated to not only reach our goal but surpass it. This feedback is fuel for our souls.

Trust me, there have been *plenty* of times in my life where I haven't gotten my way or didn't achieve what I wanted. Either I didn't get the job I desired, things did not go my way in a competition, a project didn't turn out as planned, or a certain goal was way overshot—yep . . . *way* overshot. These things happen to *everyone*; no one is immune from these hurdles.

What separates those who fail from those who achieve greatness is the reluctance to accept that event as failure. I believe that if you continue to do what you know you can, eventually, on a long enough timeline, you will achieve what you once thought was impossible. Most people fail because they give up on their goals. Giving up in my life is simply *not* an option, ever.

My journey to being a relentless rebel started early. When I was nine years old growing up in Lynchburg, Virginia, I wanted very much to play baseball rather than girls' softball—it wasn't to make a gender statement but because a baseball fit better in my small hand. The boy's league I tried to join said I couldn't play. Now, my mother doesn't take any shit from anyone, and she let them know she would be at their office Monday morning with a camera crew so they could explain why they were keeping me from playing on the league. Next thing I knew, I was approved to play baseball, and it turned out that I was pretty good at it. I held my own with the boys, and even hit a couple of home runs! I saw how powerful it was to challenge the masses who want to tell you no or hold you back.

When I first dipped my toes in fitness as an adult, I was told that I would never be an athlete. I was too scrawny, too underweight, too borderline anorexic, too much of a weakling. At the time, I was surrounded by negative people who didn't understand me or why I was training. I cared what they thought about me, sure—but not as much as I cared about my training and myself. My joy in training wasn't theirs, and I finally broke away from their negative messages. I stuck with my training and fell in love with lifting heavy weights. It took practice, discipline, and dedication to build strength. Today I'm reminded of how far I've come—and can still go.

In 2010, after I'd been in CrossFit for a while, a friend tried to get me to compete in my first CrossFit Games. These are athletic competitions in which you undergo a variety of tough athletic events that include Olympic lifting, running, powerlifting, rowing, swimming, and more. I was freaked out by the thought of competing. I hadn't yet consider myself an athlete, although I had been training like one for years.

Other friends had discouraged me, telling me that I was too small or not strong enough, or that other girls were faster than I was. I took offense at that, but also worried that they might be right. Their words weighed heavily on me and were hard to push aside. But something deep down inside me told me I could do it, because I was good at what I did.

Then a new friend encouraged me to sign up. He told me to have fun and enjoy the process. I listened to him, but I really listened to my heart. I really did want to compete. I really did want to be an athlete. And I really did want to kick some ass on a competition floor. So I entered, and out of sixty-three female contestants, I took fifth place in the sectionals and twentieth at the regionals—and was proud of it. I have competed in the CrossFit Games Open ever since then, returning to regionals four times and the Games twice, not to mention countless smaller competitions.

The more immersed I got in CrossFit, the more I explored the possibility of taking my career in a new direction. I already owned a CrossFit gym, but I wanted to make an even better living from being an athlete—with books, seminars, teaching health and wellness, and more. Even after I had been successful in opening and running a gym as well as competing, naysayers told me I could never do all these extra endeavors, but I did them all. Now I love it when someone tells me I can't or shouldn't do something, because it only fuels my fire to achieve what they perceive as impossible.

When you're mentally tough, you have the power to do whatever you put your mind to. I know, it sounds so clichéd! But it is true. You become a relentless rebel because you have a strong mental tenacity that defies what lesser minds believe. Your mental state controls the rest of your being. It's your hard drive for life.

To this day, I'm still told no. Often it takes the form of merciless criticism in social media. They'll say, "She's too muscular" or "She needs boobs." It's so easy to criticize someone without realizing that those you are finding fault with are actually people with feelings. It's really sad that people can be so passionate about something behind the security of their computer, but they would never tell you to your face. It may not be their personal choice to have a body that looks like mine. That's fine. No one has to approve of it, nor do they have to like it. It should be a lot easier to compliment someone and just be inspired by what they're doing. I want my body to help women see their own bodies differently—to see that a woman can be feminine and strong and beautiful.

Through these experiences, I ultimately shifted my thinking from allowing others to define me to asking myself, "Why *not* me?" Over time, with that mentality, I became the exception. I rebelled against the skeptics—all those naysayers, those people who didn't believe I could do things—and used them as my inspiration to go out there and show them what I'm made of. That's what a badass does!

No matter what you set out to do, there will always be doubters. But this is a positive sign. It means that you're setting yourself up to do something amazing and become the exception! So dare to push your potential.

At the same time, we don't want to be overly influenced by naysayers and their negativity—you know, go out and do things just because people say we can't. That becomes just as unreasonable as their naysaying. I prefer to be motivated by my own internal drive—by a sense of my purpose in life and what is possible for me. I look at what's important to me, and maybe someone sees my hopes and dreams as impossible or improbable, but I can't let that squash them. The next time you find yourself up against these forces, think of the word *impossible*. Broken down, it really means "I'm possible!"

Understand, too, that change frightens most people. To many, it is especially frightening to watch someone else have the courage to chase their dreams. Why? Because it eliminates their excuse for not doing so. It's much easier for them to try to talk you out of your change than to act on their own dream. Don't let someone

Are You a Relentless Rebel?

Do you take life's curve balls and face them head on? Do you stand up to naysayers or back down without a fight? Here's a quiz to help you find out. Grab a pen or pencil and mark your answers to the following questions. Be honest!

You hear that someone has been trash-talking you. How do you respond?

A. I rise above it. Trash-talking is at the expense of their character, not mine.

B. I send that person an angry text message. Two can play the trash-talking game.

C. I feel depressed that anyone would trash-talk me.

Which phrase are you most likely to overhear being said about you?

A. She is so inspiring; I'd like to get to know her better.

B. What a crazy chick.

C. I don't know how to read her. Did I do something to offend her?

When you pitch a great idea at work and a coworker promptly dismisses it, you:

A. Confidently respond, "I see what you mean, but my approach is more complex than that. I'll email everyone more details to elaborate on the concept."

B. Say, "Hey, that was a put-down. I don't see you coming up with anything better."

C. Sheepishly back off: "Forget it. It was a dumb idea anyway."

How important are others' opinions to you when you're deciding on an important course of action?

A. Somewhat important.

B. Not important.

C. Very important.

When someone says no to you, what's your reaction?

A. I take it as a dare.

B. I'm pissed off.

C. I'm dejected.

SCORING

If you marked three or more A's, consider yourself a relentless rebel. You don't let naysayers or toxic people take you down. You have the confidence to follow your own path and know that it will lead to success.

If you marked three or more B's, you aren't a goody-two-shoes, but you aren't yet a relentless rebel either. You're stuck in the middle and that's totally okay! You know how to pick your battles, and you usually aim for the least amount of controversy or drama.

If you marked three or more C's, you let yourself be guided too much by other people. Learn to rely more on your own inner strength. You have it; just learn to unleash it!

else's insecurity or small thinking determine your life! You are the one who has to live with your decisions, not them.

I recognize that many of you have been beaten down by friends, family, or co-workers who try to tell you what you can't do rather than what you can. But once you make up your mind to do something, go for it. Work hard at whatever it is, with passion, enthusiasm, and focus. Stop thinking about why you can't do it or why other people won't like it or won't believe in what you're doing. It's your life, and you don't have to answer to anyone but yourself. At the end of the day, that's all that matters.

It can be very challenging to do this, especially when people who are close to you don't see your vision, understand your purpose, or support what you are doing. I have lost many, many "friends" to my pursuit of my own happiness, and I am okay with that. The people who have stayed in my small circle are the ones who see my true self and purpose and support me even if they don't understand all of it. You'll have many chances to truly live your life the way you love, but that's also the exhilarating part—you do get to live the life you love!

So stand tall and be a shining example of what you want to represent. Don't let anyone who puts down your positive lifestyle get an upper hand. Don't accept complacency as a way of life. Proudly show the results of your success and positive attitude every day. Use that power to your advantage. Let your confidence shine through all aspects of your existence, and be a relentless rebel.

For Today

TODAY'S QUOTE

I don't worry. I don't doubt. I'm daring. I'm a rebel.
—MR. T

TODAY'S AFFIRMATION

_____

_____

_____

_____

TODAY'S CHALLENGE

Sum up your character in a single flattering phrase, such as *A Real Badass! Driven to Succeed! Superhero of the World.* Write this down and place it where you can see it often.

Imagine your phrase with your picture on a huge billboard overlooking a high-traffic major highway. Hold this image in your mind and revisit it often. Place it in a space in your house or work that you see daily. Write it on your mirror, put it in your car—wherever you will see it—and *speak it aloud* whenever you see it.

Today's Mental Goal:

_____

Today's Personal Goal:

_____

Today's Spiritual Goal:

_____

MY BADASS REFLECTIONS FOR TODAY

What are you most grateful for today?

Mentally: _____

Physically: _____

Spiritually: _____

What was the biggest success for you today?

Mentally: _____

Physically: _____

Spiritually: _____

What was the biggest challenge for you today? How did you overcome it?

Mentally: _____

Physically: _____

Spiritually: _____

What can you do tomorrow to make it a better day?

Mentally: _____

Physically: _____

Spiritually: _____

CHECKLIST

☐   I completed my habit change challenges.

☐   I made healthy choices today for my mind, body, and spirit.

☐   I've expressed my gratitude for today and all it brings, good and bad.

☐   I've prepared for tomorrow and all the unknowns it might bring.

Day 8

FUEL YOURSELF FOR SUCCESS

IMAGINE YOUR LIFE if you could build your mental toughness into a tower of strength so formidable that you always achieve your goals . . . and unleash an explosion of mental energy so powerful that you can attain whatever you desire.

Impossible? Not at all. Today you're about to find out how: by fueling yourself mentally, physically, and spirituality.

FUEL YOURSELF MENTALLY

We don't do ourselves any favors by dwelling on negative thinking. After a while, those thoughts loop around in our minds and start to sound like broken records.

The circumstances in our lives are determined by our thoughts, beliefs, and behavior (including habits)—in that order. So if you try to change a behavior or habit without circling back to the ingrained thoughts and beliefs you've had over the years, you're setting yourself up for failure.

An important solution against negativity is to fuel your mind—not with nutrients, as you do with your body, but with positive thinking, inspirational stories, and useful information. Some suggestions:

- Select a book today that you can read every morning to inspire you toward being who you want to be.
- Erase worries by staying busy on projects and other positive pursuits. Worry does not disturb busy people. When you're busy, you have no time to feed your mind on any dark, distressing thoughts. Idleness is the mother of worry and anxiety.
- Consciously focus your time and attention on the things that you have in life and want in life, and less on what you don't have or don't want. Life tends to head in the direction you're facing. If you want to improve your finances, then focus on having a great financial situation rather than on your lack of money and your debts. If you want a new relationship, focus on meeting new people and forming great relationships rather than on your loneliness. The more you focus on the positive, the sooner you'll see positive results.
- Be intensely interested in your life. That way you stay excited about your career and you continue to learn. You keep up-to-date on your industry and on the latest trends and developments in your business world. You take continuing education courses that improve not only your technical skills but also your people skills. If you're genuinely interested, several traits will show through. You'll be enthusiastic, hardworking, organized, and disciplined, and you'll always be willing to try something new.
- Stimulate your creative thinking. Whether it's coming up with innovative business ideas or deciding what to serve for dinner tonight, creative thinking is an integral part of our thought life. It's one of the secrets of business success, the power behind problem solving, and a source of greater happiness.

How can you stimulate your creativity? Tap into resources such as meeting people in new creative fields, visiting museums, reading books, or traveling to new places. You can't think out of the box if you're sitting in the box.

Also, look at a challenge or problem from a different perspective. When Jonas Salk was asked about how he invented the polio vaccine, he responded, "I pictured myself as a virus or a cancer cell and tried to sense what it would be like." This is an example of *divergent thinking*, which involves the ability to come up with different solutions and alternatives to problems by looking at them from other vantage points.

Whether you're grappling with a way to solve a business problem or thinking up an idea for a great blog, just relax, close your eyes, and let your mind wander freely. You'll be surprised by the creative ideas that pop into your mind.

- Finally, fuel yourself mentally on different points of view, talk to people from different walks of life, and look for patterns of change in your conversations and travels. If you're a Republican, hang out with Democrats. If you're a young person, walk a mile in the shoes of an eighty-year-old. Invite that family from Hong Kong to dinner. Doing so will open your mind to ideas and your life to success.

FUEL YOURSELF PHYSICALLY

"How do you eat?"

I get asked that question more than any other—and I'm glad. The food you eat can energize you, empower you, and set you up for success by fueling your performance, or it can cloud your mind and sap your physical and mental energy. Choose your foods wisely, because having a nutritious diet is the foundation of great health and mental fitness.

So what should you be eating, and when, to make sure every day fuels you for success? Here's my guide to a perfect eating day (tweak it for your needs and preferences).

Morning

AFTER YOU WAKE UP. Have a protein shake, especially if you work out in the morning. It will help rehydrate your body and skin after a night's sleep, plus it supplies your body with nutrients. A perfect shake consists of 1 scoop of protein powder, 1 cup of almond milk, ½ cup of frozen berries, and a tablespoon of almond butter blended together.

DO EAT BREAKFAST. Tons of research shows that breakfast eaters are leaner, have fewer nutrient deficiencies, and have sharper thinking skills than people who go without. For those benefits and an energy boost that lasts most of the morning, choose foods high in protein and fat and low in sugar, such as eggs, whole grains, and a fresh fruit.

Midday

DO EAT A HIGH-PROTEIN LUNCH. It increases afternoon alertness and is better for satisfying your hunger. Consuming too many carbs can trigger a post-lunch dip, leaving you feeling sluggish and mentally slow.

An ideal lunch might be one or two baked chicken breasts, a broccoli/carrot medley, and water. Other good protein choices are pork loin chops, water-packed tuna, or a couple of slices of turkey deli meat, accompanied by half an avocado, sliced tomato, and sliced cucumber. The good fats in avocado help nourish your brain and enhance blood circulation—great benefits if you're feeling tense or stressed. For a healthy dessert, have a piece of fruit such as a fresh orange.

Snacking and Hydrating

DO SNACK! Again, stick to high-protein snacks, such as smaller portions of a protein, a vegetable, and maybe a piece of fruit. This combination helps maintain your blood sugar at consistent levels.

Just don't go too long without eating, or you'll experience dips in blood sugar, which cause fatigue, irritability, and a tendency to lose focus easily. Avoid snacking on too many sweets—it can result in spikes in your blood sugar and then a drop in energy levels.

Skipping meals in general can slow down the metabolic rate, enlarge fat stores, increase daytime drowsiness, and affect concentration.

DO STAY HYDRATED. Keep drinking water or other fluids amounting to at least six to eight glasses throughout the day. Water helps you digest your food and eliminate waste products, acts as a lubricant for your joints and eyes, and boosts metabolism. Dehydration disguises itself as hunger if you don't satisfy your thirst.

Late Afternoon

DO ENJOY RECOVERY SHAKES. If you work out, have a recovery shake afterward, in order to replenish protein and muscle energy depleted by the workout. My favorite recovery shake is 1 scoop of protein powder blended with 1 cup of coconut water. Coconut water is a fantastic natural "sports drink" because it replaces electrolytes lost in sweat.

Dinner

DO MORE PROTEIN! Dinner should be similar to lunch: protein, veggies, a fat, and water. For example: 3 slices of turkey meatloaf, sautéed spinach, macadamia nuts, and water. Load up on veggies, too—they're rich in antioxidants that help slash your risk of disease.

When choosing vegetables, keep your "color count" high. Eat five to six vegetables in different colors every day. Purple cabbage, red and yellow bell peppers, dark green lettuce, spinach, carrots, green beans, and pumpkin are good food choices to maximize your nutrition.

Evening

DON'T WORRY ABOUT EATING LATER IN THE EVENING. It's a myth that this causes you to get fat. In studies, volunteers who had a large meal at eight P.M.

burned up exactly the same number of calories as others who ate the same meal earlier in the day. But be sure to have breakfast shortly after waking up and some sort of lunch in the daytime. Not eating all day and indulging at dinner will absolutely sway your metabolism in a negative way.

Before bedtime, have another protein shake made with light carbs such as almond milk and berries. This combination can promote the formation of serotonin, a feel-good chemical in the brain that helps you fall asleep.

AVOID JUNK FOOD. Highly processed foods—anything with white bread or made of white flour, sugary foods and drinks, deep-fried stuff—fall seriously short of providing you with the sustained energy and variety of nutrients you need for daily activity, and for exercise.

I know you know this! Duh! But how? The best practice for me is to not buy it in the first place! Occasionally I go on a serious hunt for something sweet. I comb through all my cabinets and fridge for that one piece of chocolate that I'm hoping I left behind. But nope, it's not there—so I can't cave in to my urges for a late-night sugar fix. If I really want a sweet, then I have to actually go out and get it. To me, it's not worth the effort. If you don't want to eat it, don't buy it. This simple rule reigns supreme for me.

FUEL YOURSELF SPIRITUALLY

There's a documented scientific link between faith and mental health. People who are engaged in some sort of spiritual endeavor have a lower risk of depression, suicide, drug abuse, and alcoholism. Having a spiritual base gives you peace and hope—two feelings that promote positive emotions. So explore a form of spirituality that speaks to you—a religion, a practice like yoga or tai chi, or spiritual readings in modern or ancient texts.

Another way to fuel your spirituality is step out of yourself and help others. Volunteer for a cause you believe in. Help a friend finish a project. Serve dinner at a homeless shelter. Being selfless and charitable is, by any moral code, a good thing.

But there's also a selfish aspect: Performing acts of kindness makes you feel good, increases your happiness, improves your immune system, and forges connectedness to higher things.

Brainpower Foods

Did you know that many foods can supply all-day mental stamina, fight bad moods, and help you process information better? It's true. Take a look at the following list and find ways to incorporate these foods into your daily diet:

- **GREEN LEAFY VEGETABLES** (spinach, kale, salad veggies, and so forth) These are high in folic acid, a B vitamin important for well being.

- **EGGS:** My favorite breakfast food is loaded with choline, a B vitamin that helps the brain make a chemical called acetylcholine, which boosts memory.

- **TUNA:** This supergood protein supplies omega-3 fatty acids, which improve mood. Plus, tuna is high in an amino acid called tyrosine, which promotes clear thinking.

- **ALL FRUITS AND VEGETABLES:** Eat more of these daily to obtain antioxidants. They protect brain cells from the destructive force of free radical molecules.

- **TOMATO AND TOMATO PRODUCTS:** All are high in the mineral selenium, known to help ease depressive moods.

- **ALMONDS:** Need more mental focus throughout the day? Snack on almonds. They're high in the mineral boron, which enhances attention.

For Today

TODAY'S QUOTE

Your mind is the channel of it all. It feeds your soul, your heart, everything.
It comes from your thoughts. The kind of person you are comes from the way
you think. And it bleeds into the way you feel. If the mind is not free, then we
won't be free.
—STEPHEN MARLEY

TODAY'S AFFIRMATION

_____

_____

_____

THIS IS A THREE-PART CHALLENGE.

FIRST, FUEL YOUR MIND. Listen to an inspirational audiobook, read an inspiring book or magazine article, or meditate on empowering thoughts. Or feed your mind pictures of things you want—especially just before you go to sleep.

SECOND, FUEL YOUR BODY. Similar to the way you plan out your perfect twenty-four hours in the challenge on page 50, I want you to simply plan out a single day of eating. Then do this every day. Writing down what you will eat daily makes it happen. And don't forget to throw out the junk food! Here's a menu planner you can use.

BREAKFAST. Choose foods such as eggs, egg whites, turkey sausage, whole-grain bread or cereal, and fresh fruits.

Date:

Weight:

_____

_____

LUNCH. Choose foods such as lean proteins—tuna, poultry, deli meat, and so on—along with greens and other vegetables.

_____

_____

DINNER. Choose foods such as lean proteins—tuna, poultry, deli meat, and so on—along with greens and other vegetables, plus starchy natural carbs such as potatoes, sweet potatoes, brown rice, quinoa, or whole-grain pasta.

_____

_____

SNACKS. Good snacks include yogurt, smoothies made with nut butters, raw veggies, nuts, seeds, and fresh fruit.

_____

_____

_____

* For precise menu examples and eating plans based on particular body types and fitness goals, check out my book _The Badass Body Diet_.

FINALLY, FUEL YOUR SPIRIT. There are many ways to do so. Think about what best fits you. Ways to expand your spirituality include:

- Setting regular sessions aside for prayer, meditation, or reflection on a regular basis.
- Connecting with others and strengthening social ties by inviting a friend to lunch or joining a club where others share your interests.
- Exploring volunteer opportunities and choosing one that's right for you.
- Renewing your relationship with nature by exercising in the park or planning an outdoor vacation.
- Practicing gratitude and counting your blessings every morning.
- Participating in mind-body-spirit activities such as yoga.

Today's Mental Goal:

_____

_____

Today's Personal Goal:

_____

_____

Today's Spiritual Goal:

_____

_____

MY BADASS REFLECTIONS FOR TODAY

What are you most grateful for today?

Mentally: _____

Physically: _____

Spiritually: _____

What was the biggest success for you today?

Mentally: _____

Physically: _____

Spiritually: _____

What was the biggest challenge for you today? How did you overcome it?

Mentally: _____

Physically: _____

Spiritually: _____

What can you do tomorrow to make it a better day?

Mentally: _____

Physically: _____

Spiritually: _____

CHECKLIST

☐   I completed my habit change challenges.

☐   I made healthy choices today for my mind, body, and spirit.

☐   I've expressed my gratitude for today and all it brings, good and bad.

☐   I've prepared for tomorrow and all the unknowns it might bring.

Day 9
BE AUTHENTIC

MY LIFE HAS been about self-discovery. Every experience I've had—good or bad—has peeled away another layer of myself, allowing me to go deeper into my soul and spirit, discover who I am, and decide if that is the real me, the person I want to be.

There have been times when I've seen myself in a way I didn't like, and it upset me. I spent a substantial part of my younger years hiding my true self, and as a result falling into a self-destructive lifestyle. But that person was not necessarily who I had to be, nor was that the person who I was destined to be. Eventually I discarded my "worthless" self and discovered my true self, my authentic self, the real me. Now I'm doing me, and I'm happy with it.

Being authentic is knowing who you are and confidently expressing this to others. It means that your thoughts, actions, words, and deeds are aligned with your underlying character.

Why is being authentic important?

AUTHENTIC PEOPLE ARE COMFORTABLE IN THEIR OWN SKIN. There's nobody on Earth just like you. Learn to embrace and accept your uniqueness, your body shape, your ethnicity, your voice, your essence, and your professional style. Once you've accepted who you are, you can share what you bring to your profession, your relationships, and the world.

AUTHENTIC PEOPLE ARE NEVER FAKE. No matter what your job may be, nobody likes interacting with a fake person. You must be your true self, because if you're not, your phoniness will be obvious to others around you. So don't try to be someone else to impress others, or try to hide your true self. Because so much of your success is based on trust, it's important to be authentic and real—at work, in relationships, everywhere.

AUTHENTIC PEOPLE KNOW THEIR STRENGTHS AND LIMITATIONS. You're good at certain things, I'm good at certain things, but we suck at other stuff. Your strengths might be communication skills, leadership, or organizational ability, but perhaps you're terrible with numbers and soft skills like patience. Be honest about your limitations while identifying your strengths. Once you've done that, sell your strengths and minimize your limitations.

AUTHENTIC PEOPLE KNOW WHAT THEY WANT AND WHAT THEY DON'T WANT. They focus on what they want. I don't like negative people; therefore, I don't hang around negative people. If you don't like something, stop pursuing it. If you don't want to work nights and weekends, then don't pursue a career in the restaurant business. If you like solitary workouts, then don't join a cardio class. If you don't like partners who are loud and braggy, then don't date that type.

Focus on what you *do* want as opposed to what you don't, and you will start to attract those things to you. Be as clear as possible about what you do want. Imagine it, feel it, embrace it. Make your thoughts strong, good, and full of what you desire. Soon enough, those things will come to you.

AUTHENTIC PEOPLE REGULARLY GO "WITHIN." Analyze your life. Ask yourself: Am I afraid to join a gym because I'm embarrassed about my shape? Is stress or depression preventing me from quitting smoking or other habits? Am I in this job or relationship that my heart's not into because I'm worried about being alone or jobless or risking confrontation?

AUTHENTIC PEOPLE LIVE WITH PASSION. I love what I do, and I never feel as if I'm "going to work." My work is very rewarding to my mind and spirit. And it gives me a sense of accomplishment, meaning, and purpose to my life. That's passion. It's what breathes life into careers and into our spirit. I do not claim to have the secret to finding passion, because it is different for everyone. But if you love what you do, know you're doing the best you can possibly do, don't mind going the extra mile, are positive and believe in yourself and your abilities, then you have passion, and you are authentic.

   Becoming authentic—being true to yourself—is one of the most powerful things you can do for your mind, body, and spirit. I believe that at any point in time, you can do anything you want to do or become anything you want to be. Each day we have the opportunity to wake up and surprise ourselves. So why not make *today* the day?

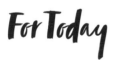

TODAY'S QUOTE

Find out who you are and be that person. That's what your soul was put on this Earth to be. Find that truth, live that truth and everything else will come.
—ELLEN DEGENERES

TODAY'S AFFIRMATION

_____

_____

_____

_____

TODAY'S CHALLENGE

Take a hard look at yourself and break with outmoded notions of who you are and what you're capable of. Be honest with yourself, and you'll be all the more satisfied for it. In your journal, answer the questions below. Be as detailed as you can.

- Am I clear about what I want to accomplish and how I want to live? If your answer is yes, write a description of what you desire to achieve and what your ideal life looks like. If it's no, why aren't you clear?
- Am I clear about who I am? If yes, describe your authentic self, including your skills, talents, and interpersonal gifts (such as compassion, encouragement, care, and so forth). If no, why aren't you clear?
- Do I downplay who I really am? If so, why?
- Can I be authentic even when it's tough? If so, how?
- Can I commit to the truth and do the right thing, rather than take the easy way out?

Today's Mental Goal:

_____

Today's Personal Goal:

_____

Today's Spiritual Goal:

_____

MY BADASS REFLECTIONS FOR TODAY

What are you most grateful for today?

Mentally: _____

Physically: _____

Spiritually: _____

What was the biggest success for you today?

Mentally: _____

Physically: _____

Spiritually: _____

What was the biggest challenge for you today? How did you overcome it?

Mentally: _____

Physically: _____

Spiritually: _____

What can you do tomorrow to make it a better day?

Mentally: _____

Physically: _____

Spiritually: _____

CHECKLIST

☐   I completed my habit change challenges.

☐   I made healthy choices today for my mind, body, and spirit.

☐   I've expressed my gratitude for today and all it brings, good and bad.

☐   I've prepared for tomorrow and all the unknowns it might bring.

Day 10

KNOW YOUR LIFE PURPOSE

I ALWAYS HEAR people talk about finding their "life purpose" or stressing to find meaning in their lives. Some of us are lucky enough to know from day 1 what we want to do in life, where we want to go, and how we want to help others. But if that's not the case for you, I'm here to tell you that it's okay.

I didn't find my purpose until my mid-twenties, after a slew of bad decisions and detours, although there were clues to my athleticism along the way—such as when I was a cheerleader and a baseball player as a kid. These clues were illuminated for only moments, similar to a flash going off in a dark room. If you had told me back then that I'd be making my living today as an athlete and entrepreneur, I would have never believed you. I would have laughed you right out of the room. Now, fifteen years later, I'm doing just that. As with me, even in the early days of your life, although likely unrecognized by you then, you had a direction. You just need to find it.

So . . . what do you do if you haven't found your life purpose yet? It's actually quite simple. Here are some tips to help you.

FIND PASSIONATE PURSUITS. Seek to discover anything that makes you feel alive, passionate, and connected to something bigger than yourself. I'm talking about whatever excites you so much that you want to keep pursuing it. These things are what give purpose and meaning to your life. Learn to recognize what ignites these positive feelings in you and embrace it!

LOOK BACK TO LOOK FORWARD. We often find our purpose in the rearview mirror. What were your dreams as a kid? What did you want to be when you grew up? What gave you joy when you were little? There's a reason that we have memories—so we can look back. As adults, most of the time we're not so good at seeing the future. When we try to look forward, our horizon looks blurry. We struggle to figure out if we are on the right track about what to do next. We look for that one thing that will give us that sense of finding our life purpose. But we need to do the opposite: look back, review our life experiences, edit out what didn't work, and recapture our dreams.

USE FEAR CONSTRUCTIVELY. Fear is excitement misplaced; it's really fuel for the soul and can ignite passion. The best things in my life have scared the shit out of me, but they are also the things that have changed the course of my life, exposing me to greater adventures, and the greatest of all adventures, discovering my life purpose and myself.

Fear also makes you focus on the task at hand. It sharpens your senses and makes you more alert. And it makes you aware of what could happen next. Let's say you've got to pitch a new product to upper management, and you're scared out of your pants. Recognize, accept, and embrace that fear, and you'll be given focus, sharpened senses, more alertness, and greater awareness as a gift. Don't fight it. Tell yourself, "Yes, I'm afraid, but I know it's making me sharper, so I'm going to do a better job at making this pitch." Once you've done this consciously a few times, the process will happen by itself. Your brain will become programmed into channeling your fear into success.

MAKE BELIEVE. There's one time of the year I really love—Christmas! After all, I was born on December 20 and named after the holiday. While pregnant with me, my mom had to stay in bed for several months to avert a miscarriage, so in gratitude, when I was born healthy, she named me Christmas Joye. I love the holiday for another reason—we get to enjoy make-believe stories about Santa and elves and others. It's not because we're deluded; instead, it's because we choose to inspire ourselves with positive and playful possibilities. When we allow ourselves to imagine, we expand the range of what we think is possible for ourselves.

So let yourself "make believe"—and imagine what you'd like to do, achieve, be, or change. Tell yourself: "I believe in me. I believe I can do anything . . . be anything, create anything, dream anything, become anything." Such make-believe fosters mental processing and decision-making, and can help create a clear vision of your life purpose.

Imagining scenes of your "dream life" helps you make better choices to lead you closer to that dream life. If you're constantly thinking about something, you'll naturally be pulled toward it. You'll emulate things that match your dream life. Eventually you'll be living that life—and dreaming of an even more amazing life.

FORMULATE A PERSONAL MISSION STATEMENT. A personal mission statement is a defining document that is the how and what of your life's purpose. Mission statements are written down, brief enough to be memorized, and reviewed regularly for progress. Unlike goals, they don't have timelines or steps to accomplish. Mission statements reflect your life's guiding philosophy—your way of being in the world. You may not be ready to create one just yet, but it's at least a good idea to start. It may even help you crystallize your life purpose.

Set aside some quiet time to ask and answer the following questions: What would you like others to remember about you? What do you want to accomplish? What kind of person do you want to be? What do you want others to experience when they come in contact with you? How will you contribute to the betterment of your profession or community or society at large?

Start with short phrases or statements about things that are near and dear to you. These are your values or beliefs that make you unique. Some of mine include: Live according to my values. Believe in myself and my abilities and let no person, situation, or factor sway me away from these. Leave a legacy, practice what I preach, and be a role model and mentor.

Also write down words to live by. These are your favorite sayings, words that define your beliefs. One of mine is *You change your thoughts, you change your world.*

There's no hurry on the way to finding your life purpose. Grandma Moses started painting masterpiece scenes of rural life at age seventy-six and continued right up until her death at age one hundred and one. A down-on-his-luck Colonel Harland Sanders turned his life around at age sixty-five when he began (with his first Social Security check!), and later built, the Kentucky Fried Chicken empire. Julia Child whipped up her first TV omelet in her fifties. Not that you have to be a late bloomer, but once you know your life purpose and are headed in the direction of your dreams, you must convert all this into specific measurable goals and then act on them with the certainty that you will achieve them.

For Today

Winners are people with definite purpose in life.
—DENIS WAITLEY

TODAY'S AFFIRMATION

_____

_____

_____

TODAY'S CHALLENGE

FIRST, I challenge you to find a playground with a swing set and swing on the swings. Spend at least ten minutes "playing" with *no phone*! This activity will help you feel alive, passionate, and connected to something bigger than yourself—and motivate you to discover other passionate pursuits on your own.

SECOND, bring the following questions to the playground. Think about these questions as you swing. Afterward, write your honest responses on a piece of paper or in your journal. Your answers will ultimately be an expression of what you are and what you are becoming.

1. What did you want to be when you grew up?
2. When you were younger, who were your heroes?

3. If money wasn't an obstacle, how would you like to spend next week?

4. If you asked good friends and loved ones to write down one compliment that each one thinks best describes you, what would be the most common compliment?

5. If you wrote a song about yourself, what would the title be?

6. What serves as the greatest inspiration for you in your daily life?

7. If you starred in a reality-TV show, how would viewers describe your personality?

8. If you could become an instant expert on one subject, what would it be?

9. If you entered a talent competition, what would you perform onstage?

10. What are the five things that make you the happiest?

11. What do you want to leave behind for your family?

Review your answers and see if you can pull out: *personal qualities* (such as friendly, intellectual, a good communicator); *dreams and ambitions*; *talents* (such as painting, singing, motivating people by public speaking, athletics, volunteering, and so forth); and *desires* (traveling, cleaning up the environment, running for political office). Review each of these. You may just discover your purpose—whether it's having a strong marriage, a fulfilling career, financial stability, a charitable commitment, or a deep spiritual connection—or you may get pretty darn close! Continue your pursuit and stay in the flow.

After you get home, write your mission statement. Think of it like a business plan and use the following template as a guide:

I [fill in your name] aspire to be a [insert personal qualities] who can use my [insert talents and/or beliefs and values] to [insert the impact you'd like to have in life] by [insert recurring actions you'll take] often, because I am supposed to [insert life purpose]. And in doing so, I live by these words: [fill in your favorite words or phrases].

Today's Mental Goal:

_____

Today's Personal Goal:

_____

Today's Spiritual Goal:

_____

MY BADASS REFLECTIONS FOR TODAY

What are you most grateful for today?

Mentally: _____

Physically: _____

Spiritually: _____

What was the biggest success for you today?

Mentally: _____

Physically: _____

Spiritually: _____

What was the biggest challenge for you today? How did you overcome it?

Mentally: _____

Physically: _____

Spiritually: _____

What can you do tomorrow to make it a better day?

Mentally: _____

Physically: _____

Spiritually: _____

CHECKLIST

☐   I completed my habit change challenges.

☐   I made healthy choices today for my mind, body, and spirit.

☐   I've expressed my gratitude for today and all it brings, good and bad.

☐   I've prepared for tomorrow and all the unknowns it might bring.

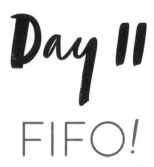

Day 11
FIFO!

IN MY WORK, I often use the term *FIFO*. It stands for (excuse my language) *figure it the fuck out*. Some of you may find this to be harsh or vulgar, but let me explain my thought process.

Any one of us can ask a question and have it answered, right? Nine times out of ten, if one of my employees, friends, or coaches doesn't know something, I or another coach, friend, or employee does. Rather than simply *giving* them the answer, I ask them to FIFO.

If we constantly spoon-feed each other information, never forcing one another to go out into the world and find the answer, we never truly reach our full potential. I mean, isn't this the whole point of Google? The resources are out there.

Figuring things out on your own takes time. It takes blood, sweat, and tears. It takes self-motivation and, above all, an eagerness to learn. Learning is at the core of FIFO, in fact, and will drive positive self-development to new heights. As the well-known author Earl Nightingale once said, "One hour per day of study will put you at the top of your field within three years. Within five years, you'll be a national authority. In seven years, you can be one of the best people in the world at what you do."

In life, there will be a lot of things you have to figure out yourself without waiting for someone else to step in. For example:

Lost your job or want to change jobs? Dust off your résumé and mobilize yourself to network. The world is full of opportunities available to you if you're resourceful enough and willing to research your options. What separates the winners from the losers is the time it takes to figure it out, get back on your feet, and get back in the ring. FIFO!

Is your lifestyle making you fat and unfit? If you're like most people, you already know enough about exercise and nutrition to be in great physical shape. You just have to cross the bridge between knowing and doing. To get there, figure out: What kind of exercise would be fun for you? What kind of healthy food would you enjoy? What kind of motivation do you need—support? an inspiring book? a workshop? Do whatever it takes to do it.

Putting something off because you don't want to face it, solve it, or do it? Kick the word *later* out of your vocabulary. You know what I mean: *later*, as in "I'll do it later." Or "I'll write that book later." Or "I know I need to get out of debt . . . I'll do it later." *Later* is a goal killer, one of the countless barriers we erect to derail our chances of success. The diet that starts "tomorrow," the job search that happens "eventually," life goals that begin "someday"—all these *laters* erect self-imposed roadblocks. FIFO and do it now! Procrastination only fuels anxiety. Get into the habit of tackling issues head-on and crossing them off your list for good. Do it, and you'll enjoy a more relaxed, productive, and healthier life.

If for some reason, you can't FIFO right away, I have a suggestion: Exercise. It's good for sharpening creativity and thinking skills. When I'm stuck and can't figure something out, I hop on the treadmill, clear my head, come back, and—bam!—I FIFO! Exercise is a way of getting what I want, a way of priming my brain for success, a secret weapon. Find your own go-to getaway and FIFO!

Whenever you discover the solutions to problems yourself, the outcome will be so much greater both internally and externally than if you were just told the answer or handed the solution. You'll feel the boost of self-worth that FIFO can bring.

Life won't always be fair. Shit happens. But you *do* have the power to create your life and change your destiny . . . if you just figure your shit out.

For Today

TODAY'S QUOTE

> *If you really want something, you can figure out how to make it happen.*
> —CHER

TODAY'S AFFIRMATION

_____

_____

_____

TODAY'S CHALLENGE

If you could go back to school for sixty days, what would you study? List your subjects below:

_____

_____

_____

Or if you don't want to hit the classroom, maybe become an apprentice working in the field in which you're interested. Where would you like to apprentice?

_____

_____

_____

What are the advantages of going back to school or becoming an apprentice? Learning and growing? Enhancing your life or the lives of your family? Increasing your financial security? Living out an unfulfilled dream? List the advantages in the space below:

_____

_____

_____

Where could you reasonably obtain this additional education? Online learning programs? Your local community center? At a nearby college or university?

Go for it—it's never too late!

Today's Mental Goal:

_____

Today's Personal Goal:

_____

Today's Spiritual Goal:

_____

MY BADASS REFLECTIONS FOR TODAY

What are you most grateful for today?

    Mentally: _____

    Physically: _____

    Spiritually: _____

What was the biggest success for you today?

    Mentally: _____

    Physically: _____

    Spiritually: _____

What was the biggest challenge for you today? How did you overcome it?

Mentally: _____

Physically: _____

Spiritually: _____

What can you do tomorrow to make it a better day?

Mentally: _____

Physically: _____

Spiritually: _____

CHECKLIST

☐   I completed my habit change challenges.

☐   I made healthy choices today for my mind, body, and spirit.

☐   I've expressed my gratitude for today and all it brings, good and bad.

☐   I've prepared for tomorrow and all the unknowns it might bring.

Day 12
DESCRIBE
YOUR LEGACY

IMAGINE THAT TODAY is the day of your funeral. A close friend or loved one steps up to the podium to deliver your eulogy. Over the next several minutes, that person will summarize your entire life and legacy.

What do you suppose this person will say? Will he or she recite only generalities? Or will the audience be so moved by the story of your life that they will momentarily forget their grief?

I have a challenge for you: If you want to leave a legacy, sit down and write your eulogy or even your obituary. How do you want to be remembered?

I include a work sheet for this in today's challenge, but here's a general overview.

Take out your journal and start by just recording the facts. Then write out how you think others might positively describe you: *She was always there for me. He was a wonderful dad who really understood his children. She spent countless hours volunteering her time.*

Then write down whatever you'd want the speaker to say. Put down on paper every last bit—little stories and scenes from your life; the nuggets of wisdom you shared; your acts of kindness and generosity; your accomplishments. Include the high points of your life, your most memorable achievements.

As you write, try to find more meaningful ways to define your life than *he was a Broncos fan* or *she loved to ski.* You want it to be about your character: how you did useful things and were a good partner and an exceptional friend.

Because you know yourself better than anyone else, there's probably no one better qualified to write these things.

Take a critical look at what you've written. Does it truly summarize your life? Are there hopes and dreams that remain unfulfilled? By writing your eulogy, you'll begin to see what truly matters—the examples you set, the goals you achieved, and the values you live by. All of these things have a positive impact on others that will endure beyond your lifetime.

I did this exercise myself. When I wrote it, I realized that much of what I do and spend my time worrying about is inconsequential. This forced me to realize that my time is limited, so maybe I need to change the way I'm spending some of it.

If the idea of an obituary or eulogy feels too gloomy, imagine your ninetieth or hundredth birthday party. Who will be there? What do you want them to say about you as they toast your birthday?

Your toast, eulogy, or obituary will reflect the legacy you want to leave. So what do you want it to be? How do you want to be remembered by those whose lives you touch?

Do this now while you have the chance to make it a reality. Then start living the way you really want to be remembered.

For Today

TODAY'S QUOTE

*The greatest legacy one can pass on to one's children and grandchildren
is not money or other material things accumulated in one's life, but rather a
legacy of character and faith.*
—BILLY GRAHAM

TODAY'S AFFIRMATION

_____

_____

_____

TODAY'S CHALLENGE

Describe your legacy. Use this work sheet to help you get specific about your
legacy; simply fill in the blanks.

_____

_____

_____

Describe stories from your life—real-life experiences that capture your personality. Think about holiday adventures, work anecdotes, family memories, unusual attributes, instances of humor, and other stories:

_____

_____

_____

Describe your character and give examples (kindness to others and how you demonstrate it, ways you deal with difficult life challenges):

_____

_____

_____

Express the values that are important to you and the ways you achieve your goals in life:

_____

_____

_____

Write down what family means to you, the love you have shared in good times and bad:

_____

_____

_____

Highlight your memorable accomplishments, special knowledge, skills, or capabilities:

_____

_____

_____

Describe the places you like to visit and why:

_____

_____

_____

Give unique milestones and historical events of your life:

_____

_____

_____

Record your favorite quotes or poems or passages of inspiration:

_____

_____

_____

List three words that sum up your life:

_____

_____

_____

Use this information to create your obituary or eulogy or mini-biography. Use the third person ("she was") rather than the first person ("I was").

Go over what you've written about yourself. Are you living up to your legacy? Where do you need to improve? What do you need to add to your life to make it reflect the legacy you'd like to leave?

Then save it. Put it in a lockbox to read again in five, ten, or thirty years!

Today's Mental Goal:

_____

Today's Personal Goal:

_____

Today's Spiritual Goal:

_____

MY BADASS REFLECTIONS FOR TODAY

What are you most grateful for today?

Mentally: _____

Physically: _____

Spiritually: _____

What was the biggest success for you today?

Mentally: _____

Physically: _____

Spiritually: _____

What was the biggest challenge for you today? How did you overcome it?

Mentally: _____

Physically: _____

Spiritually: _____

What can you do tomorrow to make it a better day?

Mentally: _____

Physically: _____

Spiritually: _____

CHECKLIST

☐   I completed my habit change challenges.

☐   I made healthy choices today for my mind, body, and spirit.

☐   I've expressed my gratitude for today and all it brings, good and bad.

☐   I've prepared for tomorrow and all the unknowns it might bring.

Day 13

LAYER IN CHANGE

CHANGE IS HARD. Really hard. I bet you know this. Maybe you've had a bad habit for years that you've tried to change: smoking, overeating, abusing alcohol, living a sedentary life. Research shows that most of us have an extremely tough time changing even a single habit. We stink at it.

When I decided to quit smoking at age twenty-two, it was a struggle. Smoking was a part of me. Cigarettes were my friend, my constant, my reassurance, my shoulder to cry on, and my supporter. I would panic if I thought I didn't have my smokes. I'd fish through my drawers like a maniac, looking for a spare cigarette. Anytime I walked by someone who was smoking, I would breathe in the second-hand smoke, happy to get a little hit of my poison.

But eventually I did quit. Now I loathe the tiniest whiff of cigarette smoke.

I did it by *layering in changes* rather than going the cold-turkey route—which never helped me quit. Here's how layering worked for me:

I prepared myself for the big quit day—my personal "Q Day." To start with, I gave myself three months to prepare. Yep, three whole months! What I was doing in that time was not cherishing my last cigarettes but mentally preparing for the toughness of quitting and getting myself excited for the possibilities to come after I quit. I knew jumping in headfirst with no preparation wouldn't lead me to long-term success.

Next, I committed to a *by when* date. I set a date to quit and would celebrate that day!

During this period I was working in Iraq. I shared my plan with my friends and coworkers there. This helped create accountability for my actions. I asked for their support and they gave it. I even told the PX (the military camp store) that I was quitting and to not sell me cigarettes after a certain date. Most people were super supportive, except maybe the die-hard smokers. I found it was best to not hang around them too much. When you're trying to kick a bad habit, you've got to surround yourself with people who will lift you up, not pull you down.

I also slowed down my smoking. I made a schedule for my smoke breaks, allotting myself only a certain number of cigarettes, or even only half of one instead of as many as I wanted.

I next traded out my smoke breaks for walking breaks. I actually was upset that smokers got to go outside more, since we couldn't smoke inside. Because I wasn't smoking as much and I still wanted to take breaks, I would grab a friend and walk around the camp, planning our vacations and projects.

By the time my Q Day arrived, I was ready for the positive change. I knew it would be hard, but I had implemented positive changes to help combat it and they worked.

Did I relapse? Sure. Did I give up? No. I just kept taking my tiny daily steps. Each little step I took in the direction of quitting brought better outcomes—from feeling better to breathing better—plus the confidence that comes with those results. I was becoming more active thanks to CrossFit; ultimately my addiction to smoking was replaced by a positive addiction to working out. I discovered that I could execute *anything* small and build big from there.

Here's where I can come to your rescue. You can overcome any bad habit if you layer in small, easy steps.

My client Miranda is another good example. She was interested in CrossFit, which is how she found her way to me.

Miranda was forty-four and overweight, with a fasting blood sugar level of 109 (prediabetic). In my mind, I could see her losing thirty pounds, doing forty-pound curls, and avoiding diabetes.

But Miranda was overwhelmed. She worked full-time and was married with three kids. She visualized a starvation diet and sweating in the gym until she dropped. She visualized laundry undone, family unfed, groceries not bought, and no time for herself. Still, there had to be a way for fitness to become a part of her life.

So how could I help her? How could we get on the same page?

I taught her how to layer in changes. I had her start with just a change at breakfast: She committed to eating a healthy morning meal. Once she nailed her breakfasts, I had her move on to healthy lunches, then dinners. Miranda's nutritional change plan looked like this:

WEEK 1: Eat a nutritious breakfast all week.
WEEK 2: Eat a nutritious breakfast and lunch all week.
WEEK 3: Eat a nutritious breakfast, lunch, and dinner all week.

One change at a time, one meal at a time—that's layering. It gave Miranda small wins, and her confidence grew.

Miranda took the same approach to exercise. I told her she didn't have to go to the gym every day. In fact, in the beginning, she didn't even have to go at all. I showed her some exercises she could do in her office three times a week: crunches and push-ups.

At first it was tough. But once a few crunches and push-ups got easy, she started doing ten. When doing ten became really easy, Miranda increased her repetitions to fifteen. Fifteen became habitual, and soon she was doing twenty-five or more every time.

After two weeks, I had her bring some light weights to her office and do an easy dumbbell routine. At the end of one month, she felt so good that she was ready to commit to a CrossFit workout three days a week. She has been going strong ever since. And yes, she is doing forty-pound curls—and more—and is thirty pounds lighter, with no blood sugar problems.

An important component to Miranda's success—and yours—is layering in enough of the right decisions. Let's say you want to lose weight. What would be some changes you could layer in? Here are some examples from a study conducted in New York City in 2015 that helped 574 adults lose weight and keep it off:

- Want to automatically reduce the amount of food you eat? Use smaller plates for main meals. Resign from the clean-plate club, too. Leave some food on your plate at meals.
- Need more fruits and veggies in your diet? Employ the *half-plate rule*. When you eat dinner, half your plate should be veggies and/or fruit; the other half should be protein and starch.
- Can't stop high-calorie snacking? Put snack food out of sight or in a place that's hard to reach. Or use the fruit-before-snack rule. Before snacking, you must eat a piece of fresh fruit first. This helps you cut back on eating fattening snack foods. Along the same lines, choose a piece of fruit when you're craving a slice or two of bread.
- Do you eat mindlessly, stuffing yourself in the process? Don't eat while your TV is on.
- Want to feel full most of the day? Eat a healthy breakfast every morning. Regular breakfast eaters do not overeat later in the day.
- Need to break that soda habit? Use the equal-water rule: Drink 12 ounces of water for every can or glass of soft drink you have.
- Gaining too much weight from eating out? Eat your main meal at home at least six days a week.

Also, if you really want to make the new, positive habit stick, choose prompts for your tiny changes. This means selecting an existing routine in your life to act as a trigger for your new behavior. For example, as soon as the phone rings, I answer it, and I start walking around or do one-legged squats. So when I take calls, I'm working out. I'm on the phone a lot each day, and now it's a habit that I probably can't stop.

The key is to evaluate which routine is the right prompt for your small, simple behavior. Maybe you need to drink more water every day, but it's not a habit for you yet. Tie drinking water to meals and snacks. Every time you eat, have a tall glass of water. Eating is your prompt to drink more water.

Prompts will be different for everyone, but the formula for your new behavior should complete the following sentence: *When I* [routine], *I will* [tiny behavior change].

So layer in small changes every day. Tie them to prompts. Little by little, as you do these things, you will start seeing progress. Once you experience a few small wins, taking bigger steps becomes easier.

For Today

TODAY'S QUOTE

I finished high school, moved to Nashville for college,
and set out to break into the music business. Every night when
I called home with news of my experiences, my mom and dad
would encourage me to keep taking those small steps.
—TRISHA YEARWOOD

TODAY'S AFFIRMATION

_____

_____

_____

TODAY'S CHALLENGE

FIFO some small changes. Check off any of the following small changes you'll
agree to try today . . . and in the days to come:

- ☐ I will eat a healthy breakfast with clean foods.
- ☐ I will drink more water.
- ☐ I will eat one salad.
- ☐ I will not use my credit card.
- ☐ I will spend five minutes meditating on my positive points.
- ☐ I will try one new vegetable.
- ☐ I will avoid alcohol.
- ☐ I will not smoke or take a harmful drug.
- ☐ I will not aimlessly surf the Internet or look at Facebook.
- ☐ I will try a new type of exercise.

Which of these small changes were the easiest to make—and why? How can
you encourage yourself to layer in these changes for good? Create an action
plan here:

_____

_____

_____

How did you feel after successfully making one or more of these small changes? Empowered? More confident? Energized? Hopeful? Describe your feelings below or in your journal:

_____

_____

Today's Mental Goal:

_____

Today's Personal Goal:

_____

Today's Spiritual Goal:

_____

MY BADASS REFLECTIONS FOR TODAY

What are you most grateful for today?

Mentally: _____

Physically: _____

Spiritually: _____

What was the biggest success for you today?

Mentally: _____

Physically: _____

Spiritually: _____

What was the biggest challenge for you today? How did you overcome it?

Mentally: _____

Physically: _____

Spiritually: _____

What can you do tomorrow to make it a better day?

Mentally: _____

Physically: _____

Spiritually: _____

CHECKLIST

☐ I completed my habit change challenges.

☐ I made healthy choices today for my mind, body, and spirit.

☐ I've expressed my gratitude for today and all it brings, good and bad.

☐ I've prepared for tomorrow and all the unknowns it might bring.

Day 14
ROCK YOUR VICTORIES

"OLD HABITS DIE hard." You've heard that saying a hundred times. One reason that they die so freakin' hard is dopamine, a chemical in the brain that gets us hooked on everything from food to cigarettes to shopping to sex.

While I have no professional credentials as a psychologist or brain expert, I do know a thing or two about dopamine. It makes you crave things. And it drives you to get them, whether they're good for you or not.

Here's what happens. First, you experience something that gives you pleasure (say, a slice of cheesecake); eating it churns out dopamine in your brain. Some of that dopamine makes a beeline to a region of your brain where memories are formed. There it creates a memory linking that cheesecake with the reward of pleasure. Whenever you're exposed to something that gives you a pleasure memory (such as cheesecake), you think, "That's bad for me, I shouldn't," but your brain registers *Yippee, dopamine rush!*

Second, in addition to forming memories, dopamine regulates the areas of the brain responsible for desire, decision-making, and motivation. So once you encounter cheesecake again, your brain produces a flood of dopamine that makes you want cheesecake. After a few delectable bites, your brain releases even more dopamine, reinforcing the memory that made cheesecake so desirable to begin with. The pleasurable sensations of eating cheesecake get etched into your brain. And the more you do something that rewards you, the more dopamine makes sure you do it again.

It's a really crazy cycle, but it is one of the ways that habits, good or bad, get etched in the brain. And it's true for any behavior that gives you a reward: Orgasms cause a dopamine rush. So does winning the jackpot when you gamble, doing cocaine or meth, smoking, drinking, and so on. Dopamine is the brain's reward system.

Okay, so how do you get yourself hooked on something that may not exactly be pleasure-producing for you, such as eating salads and broccoli or doing push-ups? Is there some way to trick the dopamine system to crave stuff that's good for us?

Yes! The secret is to create meaningful rewards for yourself. For making it to the gym all week, you could treat yourself to a pedicure or a new exercise outfit. For every month you stay away from alcohol, reward yourself with a ticket to a great concert.

Giving yourself rewards for a behavior engages the dopamine system so your brain links the positive outcome with it, which in turn helps crystallize positive habits.

But the new gratification won't necessarily kick in if the reward doesn't materialize soon enough—which is why we must reward and reinforce ourselves quickly and regularly for positive actions. Frankly, I think rewards should come at every hour of every day. We badasses deserve it, don't we?

After you eat a healthy meal, reward yourself by reading a little from a favorite book or just sitting quietly with your eyes closed. Immediate rewards are important for keeping up your motivation and acknowledging all the small steps and integrating this new habit or new way of being into yourself.

Whatever positive habit you're trying to create—whether it's ditching soda for water or getting through the day without overspending—have a reward system in place to help you celebrate your achievements. (By the way: This doesn't mean eating junk food or a box of chocolates or having a smoke or a pitcher of margaritas! If you keep justifying that cigarette or cocktail to yourself as a "stress reliever" or believe you "deserve" that candy bar, nothing's going to change.)

Instead, celebrate your success by treating yourself to something you enjoy that doesn't contradict your resolution. Here are some great ideas for celebrating your successes:

A new outfit: Here's my favorite, since I love glamming up in new clothes and heels. There's nothing like a new outfit to perk me up when I've reached a goal. It could be a cute, sexy number to wear on the weekend, a bikini for when you get down to a goal size, or even new workout clothes so that you feel good in the gym and are motivated to reach your next goal.

Music: If you're a music lover, treat yourself to some new tunes after reaching a goal. Music is a great stress reliever, too, so you might opt to reward yourself with some relaxing music to help you through the tough days.

A different hairstyle: Are you feeling better about yourself? Great! Then consider updating or changing your hairstyle or haircut to bring out your new features. Or add some highlights or color your hair differently. As you start looking fitter, a new look is a great way to show off your success.

Manicure and pedicure: Both are terrific ways to pamper yourself after working hard on your goals. Try some bright new colors to go with your new body. If you can't afford to have it done professionally, invest in some new nail polish, along with hand and foot creams.

Massage or facial: I know CrossFit competitors who treat themselves to a facial or a soothing massage every time they finish a competition. These are great rewards that renew body and spirit—plus have an antiaging effect.

Your rewards should be things that motivate you to keep going. They should also make all of your hard work and accomplishments worthwhile. Kicking bad habits and getting in great shape can be challenging, but rewarding yourself can make it much more fun.

For Today

TODAY'S QUOTE

*The more you praise and celebrate your life, the more there is in life to
celebrate.*
—OPRAH WINFREY

TODAY'S AFFIRMATION

_____

_____

_____

TODAY'S CHALLENGE

Put thirty five-dollar bills in a jar. Each day that you don't work out (or
accomplish another important goal), throw a bill in the garbage disposal and
grind it up. You're not allowed to give it to your kids or someone that needs it.
Doing a negative action with the money will motivate you to stick to what you
plan. If you were allowed to give it to someone who needs it, that would still
be a positive reward for not completing your task. Yes, this is a lot of cash but
it *has* to be. It needs to be something that hits you in the wallet or it won't be
effective. At the end of the month, use the money for a new workout outfit, or
treat yourself to something that you normally wouldn't do. So put your wallet
where your mouth is.

Today's Mental Goal:

_____

Today's Personal Goal:

_____

Today's Spiritual Goal:

_____

MY BADASS REFLECTIONS FOR TODAY

What are you most grateful for today?

Mentally: _____

Physically: _____

Spiritually: _____

What was the biggest success for you today?

Mentally: _____

Physically: _____

Spiritually: _____

What was the biggest challenge for you today? How did you overcome it?

Mentally: _____

Physically: _____

Spiritually: _____

What can you do tomorrow to make it a better day?

Mentally: _____

Physically: _____

Spiritually: _____

CHECKLIST

☐   I completed my habit change challenges.

☐   I made healthy choices today for my mind, body, and spirit.

☐   I've expressed my gratitude for today and all it brings, good and bad.

☐   I've prepared for tomorrow and all the unknowns it might bring.

Day 15
ELIMINATE EXCUSES

DO YOU EVER wonder why, despite trying, you just aren't getting the results you want in life? Maybe you've been trying to get promoted; improve your relationship; get fit; enhance your self-confidence; save more money; be more organized; or a hundred other worthwhile self-improvements. You've put energy into making these important changes, but you just aren't making headway.

What's holding you back?

I bet it's because you're making excuses.

I understand making excuses. I hid behind excuses when I refused to stop smoking, drinking, and partying. I needed my crutches, I'd tell myself. I was having too much fun, I enjoyed what I was doing, I'd say. It took a while, but I gave up the luxury of excuses once I identified my bad habits as obstacles to living a long, healthy life—which I came to desire more than anything. As a result of this hard look, I was able to change my thinking, which helped me change my behavior. Making excuses is not in the badass vocabulary!

There are thousands of excuses for not getting where you want to be in life. I've boiled them down to five. So, excuse makers, take heart. I've got ideas to get you to eliminate excuses and keep you motivated.

Excuse 1: It's not my fault.

When it comes to excuses, there are two types of people in the world: the whiners and the winners. Whiners put the blame on external factors for the results of their present life. For example, a whiner says, "I can't get ahead financially because my employer won't give me a raise." Everything is always someone else's fault. Whiners have low self-worth and low self-confidence, and are often fearful of taking action.

Winners, on the other hand, learn from their past and take responsibility to change their lives. For example, a winner says, "I'm going to work harder at my job, maybe start a business on the side, and earn and raise the extra money I need to increase my income." Winners are accountable for their actions; they do not blame others. They know that they have the power to change their lives and are willing to work hard—on their own steam.

You can create the best life possible with what you have and with what you are willing to work for. Yes, you'll face adversity, but if you press on, you will make it. At all costs, take yourself out of the whiner mindset and be one of the winners.

Excuse 2: I don't have time.

This one is probably the most used excuse, but it's also the lamest. Yours isn't a problem of time management but of self-management. If you have time to watch three to four hours of Netflix on your iPad or TV every day, you have time to work on your goals.

I got rid of cable TV for years because I found myself sucked into television shows and not working on things that would enhance the quality of my life. Did I want to just sit and watch TV and not do the work that I knew I needed to? Yes. On the one hand, I wanted to be lazy and mindless, but on the other, I wanted something better for my life. I knew that not having cable would be boring sometimes, but without it, I'd be forced to concentrate on my goals. So I created an environment that allowed me to do that.

I still have to exercise discipline toward TV, however. I create accountability checks to keep me on track so that I manage my time wisely. For example, if I want to take the day off, I make sure I get all my work done. That way I'm not stressed and can enjoy the time off, knowing that there's not a pile of unfinished business sitting around.

Do you know how you actually spend your time? Try documenting it for a few days. Record each and every thing you do and how long you do it for. You'll be shocked by the amount of time you waste by mindlessly surfing the Internet and watching TV. Transform those times into opportunities and say adios to the time excuse.

We all have the time, as long as we manage tasks, projects, people, and schedules to maximize our efficiency.

Excuse 3: I don't have the money.

A lot of people throw out this excuse. Yes, money can be an obstacle, but highly successful people see lack of money as a barrier to be overcome. They set business goals and create business plans to achieve those goals. They start where they are instead of wishing they were someplace else. They persevere against all odds. In 1980, John Paul DeJoria (who was then living in his car) teamed up with Paul Mitchell (a hairdresser) to pool their names and energy to found a company, John Paul Mitchell Systems, selling shampoos and conditioners. They started the business with only $700. Today the company is worldwide and worth billions.

In my line of work, I hear people say all the time, "I can't afford to work out or join a gym." You don't need one dime to work out. Not even one shiny little penny. Get your body outside and go for a walk. Put a mat down on the floor and do some crunches, leg lifts, squats, and lunges while you're watching TV. There are thousands of videos on YouTube you can watch for *free*! Money is the last thing you need to be fit.

If you do have some spare cash, consider purchasing some home fitness gear. For as little as fifty bucks or less, you can invest in some great home exercise toys, such as resistance bands and exercise balls, that will work your body and keep exercise fun. Or for strength training at home, use household items like heavy books or your own body weight to challenge major muscle groups.

The affordability excuse just doesn't wash with me. It stops you from taking initiative and using your badass qualities such as creativity and determination. You're the primary driver of your income—not your experience, degree, or employer. I won't say those factors have no influence, but they're neither limitations nor absolutes in dictating your income. Take full ownership of your earning potential.

Excuse 4: I'm too tired.

No, you may just be lazy. The only way you're going to get anywhere is to get off your butt and make things happen. In physics, Newton's first law of motion states that a body in motion tends to remain in motion, while a body at rest tends to remain at rest. In our lives, inertia—the tendency not to take action—is a real obstacle to success. You'll never get very far along your professional, financial, or health path. Then, before you know it, you realize that you could have accomplished so much more if only you had been willing to take action. Conversely, a body and mind in motion gets things done, and advances your goals.

One more consideration: Feeling tired can often be the result of other issues: dehydration, lack of protein, and excess dietary sugar. Make sure you eat clean and keep your body well watered.

Excuse 5: I'm too old.

Nice try. Like most things, age is a state of mind. You are as old as you think you are, and you act accordingly. This projection is what everyone sees and feels from you. I have seen eighty-year-olds act more vivacious, youthful, and energetic than most eighteen-year-olds. Age is not the limitation; your attitude about age is.

It's never too early or too late to do something you've always wanted to do. If you're in your youth, you bring mental flexibility and a fresh perspective to the table. If you're more mature, you have an edge with experience and wisdom.

Because I'm a CrossFit trainer, I've got to add that you're never too old to exercise, either! My mother started doing CrossFit in her fifties. Physical activity boosts your energy level, helps you burn body fat, alleviates stress, postpones aging, and renews your confidence.

Also, if you want to be ageless and perhaps live longer, you've got to exercise. It has been shown to extend an individual's life-span by as much as five years. A small but recent study discovered that exercise of moderate intensity may slow down the aging of our cells. As we get older and our cells divide over and over again, our telomeres, the protective caps on the ends of our chromosomes, get shorter. To learn how exercise affects telomeres, scientists took muscle biopsies and blood samples from ten volunteers before and after they rode 45 minutes on stationary bicycles. The researchers observed that exercising increased levels of a molecule that protects telomeres, ultimately slowing down how quickly they lose their length. Pretty cool stuff: Exercise slows aging at the cellular level. You could easily gain five or more years to set and attain even more life goals.

Finally, I'll add some overarching advice: Whenever you start making excuses, let your thoughts continue until you picture what the end result will be (financial issues; dead-end job; soft, flabby, tired body!) The more clearly you can visualize the consequences of your actions, the greater the chance you'll make better decisions.

For Today

Ninety-nine percent of the failures come from people who have the habit of making excuses.
—GEORGE WASHINGTON CARVER

TODAY'S AFFIRMATION

_____

_____

_____

TODAY'S CHALLENGE

In the space below, write down three excuses you use in your life to not pursue a successful lifestyle:

Excuse 1: _____

Excuse 2: _____

Excuse 3: _____

In the space below, reflect and write down how your making of excuses has prevented you from living up to your potential and achieving the dreams you imagine:

_____

_____

Action Plan for Excuse 1: _____

Action Plan for Excuse 2: _____

Action Plan for Excuse 3: _____

Today's Mental Goal:

_____

Today's Personal Goal:

_____

Today's Spiritual Goal:

_____

MY BADASS REFLECTIONS FOR TODAY

What are you most grateful for today?

Mentally: _____

Physically: _____

Spiritually: _____

What was the biggest success for you today?

Mentally: _____

Physically: _____

Spiritually: _____

What was the biggest challenge for you today? How did you overcome it?

Mentally: _____

Physically: _____

Spiritually: _____

What can you do tomorrow to make it a better day?

Mentally: _____

Physically: _____

Spiritually: _____

CHECKLIST

☐   I completed my habit change challenges.

☐   I made healthy choices today for my mind, body, and spirit.

☐   I've expressed my gratitude for today and all it brings, good and bad.

☐   I've prepared for tomorrow and all the unknowns it might bring.

Day 16

PUT IN THE
EFFORT

WHILE I WAS writing this book, the 2016 Summer Olympics in Rio were winding down. I like watching the Olympics because they showcase the possibilities we all have to push the boundaries of human potential. I got to thinking, "What really makes those athletes so special?"

Training for the Olympics is a full-time job. Olympians don't just bike, swim, or run for an hour after working a regular job. They train many hours a day. And that's just to get ready for the competition at hand. It takes at least four to eight years of training to be in good enough shape to compete on an international level. These athletes map out their training in increments of years, not days. It's not just a matter of toughing it out. They've developed near-superhuman lung and heart capacity, plus amazing muscular strength.

I realize you're not prepared to give up your entire life for a shot at a little piece of medal on a ribbon (unless you want to!), but I think there's a lot we can learn from the Olympians about putting in the effort to be the very best we can be. How? By approaching your life with the single-minded focus of a world-class athlete.

Great athletes have dreams and goals—both fueled by a burning desire to win. They constantly dwell on these goals, so that's why they eventually achieve them. But none of this comes without hard work and effort. Michael Phelps, the greatest Olympian ever with twenty-eight medals (including twenty-three gold), was known for his intense training and consistent prerace routine, all geared to get him to his goals. Not everyone needs to hit the Michael Phelps level of dedication. But we can learn from his commitment to achieving his goals and putting in the effort to attain them.

Athletes usually have someone as an inspiration and strive to become as great as or even greater than that idol. Find an idol or hero of your own. Draw inspiration from their effort and emulate it. I'm moved by the story of Glenn Cunningham, once considered the world's fastest human being. When he was a boy, his legs were badly injured in a fire, and his doctor wanted to amputate them. Thankfully that didn't happen, but the burns left his right leg almost three inches shorter than the other, and the toes on his left foot were completely burned off. Yet young Glenn was fiercely determined. He forced himself to exercise every day. Soon he threw away his crutches and started walking. And then he was running and running and running. Those legs that had been so close to being amputated carried him to a world record in the mile run. He won a silver medal in the 1500-meter run in the 1936 Olympics and competed successfully in many other running events.

Athletes are self-reflective. They look inside themselves and ask some deep questions about their performance and their life direction. They push aside negative thoughts, telling themselves, *You're a winner!* One of my favorite examples of a winning attitude is the story of Natalie du Toit, who became an internationally ranked swimmer in her native South Africa by the age of fourteen. Sadly, three years later, in 2001, she was hit by a car on her way back to school from swim practice and lost her left leg at the knee. But Natalie pressed on: She won gold medals at the 2004 Paralympic Games, as well as the Commonwealth Games. She was one of two Paralympians to compete at the 2008 Summer Olympics in Beijing, and she became the third amputee ever to qualify for the Olympics. Her motto is *Be everything you want to be.* Natalie has demonstrated to the world that if you have a winning attitude, there is no obstacle too great to overcome.

Ask yourself: What changes would you like to see, and what benefits will those changes bring to your life? Put your effort into all things positive and imagine what it would be like to get rid of the negative energy you've wasted on excuses. Positive self-talk is not the same as bragging or Pollyannaish optimism. It simply reflects a conscious effort to flood your mind with positive, nurturing, performance-enhancing thoughts that change your life for the better.

And finally, athletes exert enormous physical effort. They train hard. They practice. They show up. They go the distance—literally and figuratively.

What does your effort look like? Start assessing this aspect of your life with the quiz on page 134.

THE 10 COMMANDMENTS OF A FULL-EFFORT BADASS

If you feel like you've got to put in more effort and not sure where to start, I've developed ten effort-building principles that lead to a balanced, fulfilling, healthy life. They will help keep you on track.

1. I will remember that time is not a measurement of hard work. Putting effort into something is not reflected by long hours. The true measure of your effort is the fact that you have worked to the best of your ability to complete a goal.

I've noticed this issue most recently with my work schedule. I've been running around like a chicken with my head cut off. Yep, I said it—I admit, I utterly overworked myself. Between traveling nonstop, a million events and projects, and bigger-picture items that require attention (not to mention my personal life, my new fiancé, my dog, Fran, and my gym family), I've been spread too thin.

I've always led a fast-paced life. I don't know any other way to be—it's in my nature, in my blood. This has benefited me greatly because it's one of the few things that can't be taught. You can teach someone how to lift or how to complete a task at work, but you can't teach hard-core drive. This kind of work ethic is internal, inherent in you.

I came to the hard realization that long, fast-paced hours aren't always most effective—which is why I created this commandment and put it first. Sometimes when we're moving too quickly, we miss grand opportunities and our performance isn't anywhere near our best. If we can take the time to slow down (with our fitness movements, with our work), we can actually increase our productivity. Find yourself spinning too fast? Then consciously take the time to slow down, acknowledge the indications of stress, and adjust your schedule accordingly. You'll be amazed at how much you begin to accomplish!

2. I will follow through on my commitments. If a particular undertaking is frustrating you, write down the subsequent steps you need to take and include a specific time frame. This allows you to quickly regain your momentum when you return to the task.

3. I will work with passion. Every area of your life demands effort—on the job, at home, and in the gym. If you love what you do and how you live—in other words, you're passionate about life—your effort will be fun, more productive, and virtually stress-free.

4. I will make an effort to be courteous and kind. This is a spiritual decision with amazing benefits. You'll attract more customers and friends—and win them for life by doing good and being good. This effort may be the one thing that sets you apart from your competition.

5. I will put all my effort into going after my dreams, moving forward against obstacles, and learning from failure. This commandment is the core of a winning attitude. Winners do the things that other people won't, and that's what makes them stand out.

6. I will be motivated to learn and change for the better because I am worth the ef-

fort. Do your homework by consulting books and magazines, reading inspirational books to feed your spirit, researching successful people you admire and how they succeeded, and talking to other entrepreneurs, mentors, counselors, or experts.

7. I will apply effort to my workouts, diet, and health. The highest-performing people (think athletes!) have an unwavering desire to be the best, and are willing to put in the effort required to achieve that level of success. They work diligently toward their goals even when the results are hard to obtain. Pressure is a privilege. So if you want a killer body, work to your maximum potential. Don't put it off. Don't blow it off. That's the difference between good enough and the best you can be.

When it comes to health and fitness, your motivation should be a no-brainer; facts prove exercise and eating well can add longevity and quality of life. Your inspiration to eat healthy and to exercise could come from many different things, whether you want to fit into a pair of jeans or you have some real, substantial athletic goal. Your inspiration changes all the time.

8. I will not become complacent. Many people work really hard to be successful, yet when they reach the top, forget what got them there . . . or how to stay there. They get spoiled by success. Never let up; never stop putting in the effort. Remember what brought you success in the first place.

9. I will stay disciplined. This commandment speaks to changing bad habits and forming good ones. Your daily habits will make or break your success. Eating right, abstaining from dangerous substances, practicing spirituality, managing your life productively, and other such actions are all essential habits that require persistent and consistent effort—in other words, discipline.

10. I will live with 100 percent integrity. Never do or say anything that wouldn't make your mother, father, spouse, or children proud. Don't cause harm, violate moral codes, or damage the environment. Don't lie, insult, or cheat in pursuit of success. It just isn't worth it. This commandment is simple: If it doesn't feel right, then it probably isn't, so don't do it.

We can learn a lot from great athletes, whether we are competing in sports or engaging in demanding activities in life. We've got to hone, practice, and develop our skills over time to improve or master them. Don't place limits on yourself. You have inside you the seeds to become anything you want, even an Olympic champion.

Quiz: What's Your Life Effort?

Read the questions below and answer honestly.

1. When working on achieving my goals, I put in maximum effort and work even harder if I suffer a setback.

A. A lot
B. Often
C. Sometimes
D. Rarely
E. Never

3. I tend to do the maximum amount of work necessary to keep my boss and my team on course.

A. A lot
B. Often
C. Sometimes
D. Rarely
E. Never

2. I believe that if I work hard and apply my abilities and talents, I will be successful.

A. A lot
B. Often
C. Sometimes
D. Rarely
E. Never

4. When an unexpected event threatens or jeopardizes my goal, I set a different goal and move in a new direction.

A. A lot
B. Often
C. Sometimes
D. Rarely
E. Never

**5. When I see a strategy that works,
I want to nurture it.**

A. A lot
B. Often
C. Sometimes
D. Rarely
E. Never

6. I look for opportunities to excel.

A. A lot
B. Often
C. Sometimes
D. Rarely
E. Never

**7. I actively seek opportunities to build
wealth and/or create financial security.**

A. A lot
B. Often
C. Sometimes
D. Rarely
E. Never

**8. I feel energized after an intense workout
or after completing a project.**

A. A lot
B. Often
C. Sometimes
D. Rarely
E. Never

**9. The force that drives me to do
things is strong.**

A. A lot
B. Often
C. Sometimes
D. Rarely
E. Never

10. I consider myself self-reliant.

A. A lot
B. Often
C. Sometimes
D. Rarely
E. Never

11. I tend to be a positive thinker.

A. A lot
B. Often
C. Sometimes
D. Rarely
E. Never

**12. I enjoy setting new goals
and going after them.**

A. A lot
B. Often
C. Sometimes
D. Rarely
E. Never

(cont.)

SCORING

For each A, give yourself 5 points; for each B, 4 points; for each C, 3 points; for each D, 2 points; and for each E, 1 point. Count up your total number of points.

44 to 60 points: Great job. You are highly motivated most of the time and put in the effort to make things happen.

28 to 43 points: You're doing fairly well on effort, but could achieve more. Look for areas in your life that would benefit from more effort and motivation.

12 to 27 points: You're kind of coasting and not setting or achieving many goals. Break this harmful pattern now, and start believing in yourself again.

For Today

TODAY'S QUOTE

Continuous effort—not strength or intelligence—
is the key to unlocking our potential.
—WINSTON CHURCHILL

TODAY'S AFFIRMATION

_____

_____

_____

TODAY'S CHALLENGE

After reading through this chapter and taking my quiz, come up with strategies that can help you bump up your effort—in exercise, fitness, and life in general. Look through each of my commandments and select the one or ones you need to work out. Then list steps you can take to make those commandments a reality in your life. Take commandment 7, for instance. Maybe you need to lift heavier weights, run farther, or push yourself more often during the week.

Today's Mental Goal:

_____

_____

Today's Personal Goal:

_____

_____

Today's Spiritual Goal:

_____

_____

MY BADASS REFLECTIONS FOR TODAY

What are you most grateful for today?

Mentally: _____

Physically: _____

Spiritually: _____

What was the biggest success for you today?

Mentally: _____

Physically: _____

Spiritually: _____

What was the biggest challenge for you today? How did you overcome it?

Mentally: _____

Physically: _____

Spiritually: _____

What can you do tomorrow to make it a better day?

Mentally: _____

Physically: _____

Spiritually: _____

CHECKLIST

☐   I completed my habit change challenges.

☐   I made healthy choices today for my mind, body, and spirit.

☐   I've expressed my gratitude for today and all it brings, good and bad.

☐   I've prepared for tomorrow and all the unknowns it might bring.

Day 17
BE UNSTOPPABLE

IF YOU'VE EVER heard the fable of the two frogs in the bucket of cream, well, I'm the frog who kept kicking and flopping, refusing to give up, while the second frog stopped kicking and drowned because he thought they were doomed. As the first frog kicked like crazy, the cream was churned into butter, so he was able to climb on top of it and hop out of the bucket.

The frog lesson is clear: Even when we can't see our way out, continue kicking and trying like hell. I like to think that's the way I live. I keep trying, I stay the course, regardless of how many barriers are placed in front of me or the noes I receive. Why? Not because I'm the best or the strongest or the fastest, but because of the positive habits I've built over the years, and because of my consistency in applying those habits. I refuse to believe anything other than what I am working toward is possible. I stay constant in my pursuit of my goal.

Consistency means you're unstoppable. You stay the course—no yo-yoing between virtuous salads and "screw-it" cheesecakes in any given week, no working hard one or two days a week at something, then slouching on the couch the rest.

Right now it might seem tough to find the strength to continue to live your dreams. There will be times where you want to quit, you don't want this anymore, it is too freakin' hard, and you wonder why you even tried.

Well, guess what? That day is your defining day.

On that day, you absolutely must keep going and keep kicking—with conviction and unwavering focus on your original goals. Start talking to yourself continuously, saying, "I am unstoppable!"

Let me introduce you to Flora from Scotland, who knows how to be unstoppable against incredible odds. She emailed me after watching a live video I did on Facebook to tell me her story. Flora has bipolar depression, which is a serious mental health issue marked by up and down mood swings. One of the ways she copes and eases her depression is through fitness and exercise (go, Flora!). At five foot four, Flora once weighed 210 pounds—which didn't do much for her already messed-up moods. But she kept working at her weight and health, *consistently*, and today she weighs in at a healthy, fit 118 pounds—and she is definitely unstoppable.

Flora is living proof that consistency is another big key to success, yet it's one of the biggest struggles to achieving goals. Most people don't know how to sustain it. I do. Flora does.

If you want to be unstoppable, here are some strategies:

TAKE A DAY-BY-DAY APPROACH. Concentrate on what you have to do *today* only. Success is a daily habit, not a "once in a while, when you have time" sort of thing. Each "today" adds up—to a week, a month, two months, six months, a lifetime. Get through *that* day and you will be unstoppable.

ASK YOURSELF THE HARD QUESTIONS. Example: "Do I want to be in a low-paying job for the rest of my life?" Of course your answer is going to be no! Ask and answer those hard questions whenever you want to toss in the towel, and you *will* keep up your momentum! So for now, think about what you want, pin it down, ask yourself why you want it so badly. Your desire should be so strong that nothing is too hard, no hours are too many, no effort goes unmade, and no matter what, you keep going because you want out of the bucket.

MAKE YOUR SCHEDULE NONNEGOTIABLE. Agreeing to every commitment that comes your way may help you win a popularity contest, but it also means less time for working on your goals. Carve out a regular schedule and stick to your priorities. Don't let meeting excess family obligations, doing favors for people, or socializing keep you from achieving your goals. Don't get me wrong—there's nothing bad about these activities. It's just that they can suck up all your time if you don't manage them properly and stick to your priorities. Yes, you've got to spend time with your family; just make sure it's quality time. Helping other people is a great virtue, but don't neglect your own needs. As for socializing, it can be a great way to spend time with people who share your passions and role models from whom you can learn new or better ways of accomplishing your goals.

ADOPT A "SUCCESS" IDENTITY. Visualize yourself as a successful, positive achiever, and that's who you'll become. It's true! You'll automatically and effortlessly choose actions that support your vision and allow you to reach your life goals. Another example: If you are trying to quit smoking, keep saying to yourself, "I am a nonsmoker," and your mind will start believing you; that's when success happens. Whatever identity you choose, that's who you are and what you do.

DON'T BEAT YOURSELF UP OVER BACKSLIDING. Just start anew next time. I was once told: "We all fail, but you need to fail quickly and move on."

Approach your life this way; it's what separates the winners (like the frog who kept kicking) from the also-rans (like the frog who drowned in the cream). Once you get some momentum going, you will be unstoppable.

For Today

TODAY'S QUOTE

*Good, better, best. Never let it rest. 'Til your good
is better and your better is best.*
—SAINT JEROME

TODAY'S AFFIRMATION

_____

_____

_____

TODAY'S CHALLENGE

One way to adopt your "success identity" is to select as a role model someone (such as a high-profile businessperson) who has already achieved what you want to accomplish. This works because it helps you step away from your own way of being in the work, and encourages you to explore and adopt the values, priorities, passion, and motivation of the person you are modeling. When you do this—when you model your life after someone you admire—you begin to attract all the same things into your life as your role model exhibits. Trust me, this technique can get you to your goals faster.

Start by studying the person who you are modeling through biographies, autobiographies, and interviews. Find out his or her success secrets and the values he or she held that took that person to the top. Write down all the behaviors and qualities you find about the person; then try to incorporate as many as possible into your own life.

Today's Mental Goal:

_____

Today's Personal Goal:

_____

Today's Spiritual Goal:

_____

MY BADASS REFLECTIONS FOR TODAY

What are you most grateful for today?

Mentally: _____

Physically: _____

Spiritually: _____

What was the biggest success for you today?

Mentally: _____

Physically: _____

Spiritually: _____

What was the biggest challenge for you today? How did you overcome it?

Mentally: _____

Physically: _____

Spiritually: _____

What can you do tomorrow to make it a better day?

Mentally: _____

Physically: _____

Spiritually: _____

CHECKLIST

☐   I completed my habit change challenges.

☐   I made healthy choices today for my mind, body, and spirit.

☐   I've expressed my gratitude for today and all it brings, good and bad.

☐   I've prepared for tomorrow and all the unknowns it might bring.

Day 18
ADJUST YOUR ATTITUDE

WHAT DOES YOUR attitude say about you?

Attitude is made up of what you think, what you do, and what you feel. It's really your spirit.

With a good attitude, you can successfully deal with challenges, get past the annoying stuff, overcome obstacles, and achieve your goals. You're like a bright light, shining with optimism and positive energy. This energy sets good things into motion and allows you to see opportunity in opposition or setbacks. It creates positive thoughts and positive habits. When a devastating event happens, you'll automatically look for the good in the situation, even a new positive opportunity. The loss will make you stronger and better in the long run. You may suffer setbacks, make mistakes, or get dragged down by hard times, but you can usually weather the storm and come out on top.

With a bad attitude, you tend to complain a lot, criticize people and things frequently, and seem to carry a dark cloud over your head. Negative energy creates self-loathing and poor-me victim thinking, drains your efforts, and points you in a bad, dead-end direction.

The difference between having a good attitude or a bad attitude could make or break your day—how you feel and perform—or even affect how your whole life turns out. Your attitude sets the atmosphere for your habits and work and affects how you feel and how you perform. It's a positive tool for positive action. Your attitude reflects you.

Now that you've assessed yourself, here are some strategies for change.

CHOOSE A GOOD ATTITUDE. Attitude is a choice. You must choose to stay positive, even when you are engulfed in sadness. You have the power to see situations more positively. I learned this in 2015—a devastating year for me. My mom went through breast cancer treatment, a significant relationship ended, and I didn't perform up to par in competition. I wanted to stay sad, in bed, and not work out or be social. I wanted to quit everything and hide, but deep down, I knew that would only prolong my misery. I had to make a choice to move on, get out of bed, go to my seminars, meet up with friends, spend as much time as I could with my mom and help her through her treatments, and just generally make moves to get on with my life.

What I learned was that I needed to tell myself every morning that I'm going to display a good attitude throughout the day. This choice—this control of my attitude—renewed my self-confidence and made it unshakable. Never forgetting that you have a choice is the key to unlocking your greatness in life. Choice is powerful; use it in a positive way!

PROTECT YOUR MIND FROM ANY NEGATIVE SELF-TALK. Your mind is your number one ally when it comes to achieving your goals. You want to be in better shape, for example. Yet you still continue to think of yourself as flabby and out of shape. Stop that negativity! Reprogram your mind to think of yourself as fit, sexy, and attractive, and you'll be well on the path toward achieving those goals.

Whenever a negative thought comes to mind, immediately reject it. (Remember the rubber-band exercise from day 1!)

Attitude Quiz

Do you often have a bad attitude, or are you able to look on the positive side? Find out by taking the following quiz:

1. When you get up in the morning, you can't wait to start the day and see what it brings.

A. True
B. False

2. If something you've been planning doesn't work out, you concentrate your energy on making it work or finding ways to salvage the situation.

A. True
B. False

3. You feel that life is mostly a daily grind.

A. True
B. False

4. If there's an obstacle in the way, you figure out what you're going to do about it.

A. True
B. False

5. Your best friend becomes seriously ill. You assure her that you're there to help—with what she needs (child care, emotional support, errands, and so forth).

A. True
B. False

6. On New Year's Eve, your main thought is "Another year bites the dust."

A. True
B. False

7. You're stuck in traffic and get mad as hell.

A. True
B. False

8. In your self-talk, you tend to use positive and encouraging phrases.

A. True
B. False

(cont.)

9. You tend to worry a lot, even about things over which you have no control.

A. True

B. False

10. You tend to dwell on your weak points more than on your strong points.

A. True

B. False

11. If you get criticized, you feel depressed.

A. True

B. False

12. You usually see the worst in people.

A. True

B. False

13. When something goes wrong in your life, you tend to blame others.

A. True

B. False

14. When things get stressful, you focus on solving the situation.

A. True

B. False

15. It is easy for you to forgive people.

A. True

B. False

SCORING

Step 1. Review your answers. Count the numbers of A's and B's you selected. Record them in the box on page 153.

Step 2. Count up your points. If you scored between 60 and 75 points, you have a great attitude. You are in love with life and everything that it can bring, and you throw yourself into it 100 percent. You know how to get the most out of everything that you do.

If you scored between 55 and 30 points, you have an average attitude. You take the good and bad in life as they come, though sometimes you need to run your life with a little more positivity.

If you scored under 30 points, take stock of how you look at the world. Your tendency to be negative may block your ability to achieve your goals and get the most out of life.

Question	Your Answer (A or B)	Score	
1		If you answered A, give yourself 5 points; if you answered B, give yourself 0 points.	Your points:___
2		If you answered A, give yourself 5 points; if you answered B, give yourself 0 points.	Your points:___
3		If you answered A, give yourself 0 points; if you answered B, give yourself 5 points.	Your points:___
4		If you answered A, give yourself 5 points; if you answered B, give yourself 0 points.	Your points:___
5		If you answered A, give yourself 5 points; if you answered B, give yourself 0 points.	Your points:___
6		If you answered A, give yourself 0 points; if you answered B, give yourself 5 points.	Your points:___
7		If you answered A, give yourself 0 points; if you answered B, give yourself 5 points.	Your points:___
8		If you answered A, give yourself 0 points; if you answered B, give yourself 5 points.	Your points:___
9		If you answered A, give yourself 0 points; if you answered B, give yourself 5 points.	Your points:___
10		If you answered A, give yourself 0 points; if you answered B, give yourself 5 points.	Your points:___
11		If you answered A, give yourself 0 points; if you answered B, give yourself 5 points.	Your points:___

12		If you answered A, give yourself 0 points; if you answered B, give yourself 5 points.	Your points:___
13		If you answered A, give yourself 0 points; if you answered B, give yourself 5 points.	Your points:___
14		If you answered A, give yourself 5 points; if you answered B, give yourself 0 points.	Your points:___
15		If you answered A, give yourself 5 points; if you answered B, give yourself 0 points.	Your points:___

BE A SOLUTION-SIDE PERSON. When bad stuff comes your way, whether it's money problems, relationship issues, health challenges, or other problems, be on the lookout for answers and solutions, not scapegoats. People with negative attitudes tend to look for something or someone to blame. For example, if a negative thinker faces a particular challenge or problem, he or she may ask, "Why does this always happen to me?" Are you like that? If so, try something positive, such as "What can I do to make the situation better?"

Positive thinkers accept the situation as just a problem that must be solved, wasting very little time on blame or victimizing themselves. They get to the heart of the matter and emerge stronger than ever.

STAY IN THE MOMENT. How many times have you been there but not really there? You know—you're sitting in a meeting but focusing on what you have to do next week. Or you're at the gym, working out, but all you're thinking about is what you're going to fix your family for dinner. When I coach clients, I always emphasize that they should make sure they stay in the moment with everything they're doing, and they'll do it well.

So, staying in the moment? I believe it strengthens your positivity and lightens your life.

SMILE OFTEN. A few years ago, I came across a simple idea that has been validated in hundreds of experiments and can change your attitude, help you feel happier, and boost your confidence. Force yourself to smile, whether you feel like it or not. It will change your attitude in an instant.

Researchers have studied this phenomenon for ages, using various ways to create forced smiles on volunteers and finding that when people repeatedly forced smiles, they suddenly felt much happier and more positive. Smiling and laughing generates enthusiasm, friendliness, and goodwill. So why not smile more?

Keep a positive attitude, even when you are devastated, and it will give you the best opportunity to always find success in both your trials and your adventures.

For Today

TODAY'S QUOTE

If you change the way you look at things, the things you look at change.
—WAYNE DYER

TODAY'S AFFIRMATION

_____

_____

_____

Practice positive self-talk. Starting today, improve your attitude by using positive self-talk. Make a list of all the things you have done or now do well: jobs, sports, hobbies, and anything you are proficient at. Also include words describing your positive traits, such as *respectful*, *courteous*, *well-mannered*, *friendly*, and so forth. When you finish, read your list out loud. For example, read aloud, "I am a friend. I'm good at making sales calls, refinishing furniture, singing, and painting," or whatever you have on your list. The reason for reading the list aloud is that this act deeply etches in your subconscious mind those things that you do well. Read your list aloud just before going to sleep at night and first thing each morning. Whenever you master new things, add them to your list. Practice this exercise at night and in the morning every day, and you'll soon see a big turnaround in your attitude.

Today's Mental Goal:

_____

Today's Personal Goal:

_____

Today's Spiritual Goal:

_____

MY BADASS REFLECTIONS FOR TODAY

What are you most grateful for today?

Mentally: _____

Physically: _____

Spiritually: _____

What was the biggest success for you today?

Mentally: _____

Physically: _____

Spiritually: _____

What was the biggest challenge for you today? How did you overcome it?

Mentally: _____

Physically: _____

Spiritually: _____

What can you do tomorrow to make it a better day?

Mentally: _____

Physically: _____

Spiritually: _____

CHECKLIST

☐   I completed my habit change challenges.

☐   I made healthy choices today for my mind, body, and spirit.

☐   I've expressed my gratitude for today and all it brings, good and bad.

☐   I've prepared for tomorrow and all the unknowns it might bring.

Day 19
LEAN ON MENTORS

I NEED INSPIRATION to clean my house. Who doesn't, right? So I look at a picture of my grandmother on my mother's side, Grandma Rowland. She'd always tell me to sweep my front porch on Sunday, because this shows respect for the neighborhood and demonstrates that you take care of your home and yourself. Come housework day, I smile at Grandma Rowland, crank up some fun, fast-paced music, and open my doors and windows. Before long, I'm cleaning my house like a madwoman.

You could say that Grandma Rowland was one of my first mentors, because she was wise and I learned from her. She was a strong, caring woman who filled my life with inspiration and hope, and her lessons continue to influence me today. She taught me to work hard and do my best.

While I was working in Iraq, Jim, one of the marines, took me under his wing. He not only became my personal trainer free of charge but also turned into a great mentor. Weighing about 95 pounds at the time, I took one look at some barbells and said, "Do you think I can lift those?" He replied, "I know you can."

Jim taught me how to eat right and train hard. He taught me discipline and emphasized the importance of rest. Because I needed to build muscle and put on size, we trained intensely. I started seeing major results, and so did everyone around me. And guess what? My life began to mend as I developed both inner and physical strength. This powerful combination helped me stop my destructive habits.

A mentor is like that—someone who helps you get more from life in a positive, action-oriented way by stressing what you can do rather than what you can't. A mentor can play any number of roles—coach, motivator, cheerleader, and consultant—guiding you from where you are to where you want to be. Do you want to start a new career? Do better on your job? Build wealth? Improve your health and fitness? Reduce stress? Get a mentor!

People who use mentors are more successful than those without mentors, and that's substantiated by academic research. People who have mentors get more promotions, make more money, and have more career and job satisfaction.

Why is this? As I see it, there are three reasons. Mentors:

- Expand your awareness: A mentor can sense cracks in your knowledge, fill in the gaps, help you FIFO, and show you new ways to look at the world.
- Teach you new skills. A mentor can introduce you to new ways to do things or help you increase your capabilities.
- Show you the tools. A mentor may know a lot more about management, leadership, goal setting, personal finance, relationship success, fitness, spirituality, and other aspects of life than you do. Mentors have the tools, have mastered their use, and can show you how to apply them.

So how in the world do you go about finding a mentor?

REVIEW YOUR GOALS. I suggest going back to your goals and revisiting them. Then ask yourself, "What skills do I need to develop in order to reach my goals? What do I struggle with and what would I like to do better?"

DO A MENTOR SEARCH. Then start looking for a mentor who has those skills, through formal mentoring programs at your place of employment, at your gym, or online through an e-mentoring service. Tell everyone you can that you're looking to connect with a mentor, and get some referrals. Use social networking tools, such as LinkedIn, to help.

FIND AN INFLUENTIAL MENTOR. Make sure potential mentors hold a place of power in their industries—such as a really successful personal trainer, businessperson, entrepreneur, or leader. You want to find someone whose success you'd like to emulate. This will ensure that he or she has the skill and experience to really help you. Worth mentioning, too, is that you can cultivate mentors for different aspects of life—for example, a mentor for fitness and a mentor for business. A mentor does not have to be full service!

ASK FOR HELP. Once you've identified what you want from a mentor, the next step is approaching someone and asking for his or her time. Don't be shy. Most people are flattered to be asked to be a mentor. In reality, we all like to be asked for advice. They may say no or refer you to someone else, and that's okay. You will have learned something even from how well your approach worked.

DEFINE THE RELATIONSHIP. Make it clear that you won't be ultra-demanding, with a zillion questions, phone calls, texts, and emails—and that you'll be accountable for following through on your mentor's advice and suggestions. Bottom line: Be respectful of your mentor's time. As a mentee, think of things you can do for your mentor, too, such as providing constructive feedback, being grateful and showing it, and recommending your mentor to others in order to help push his or her business forward. If your relationship runs its course, let your mentor know how much you appreciated having him or her in your life.

BE A GOOD STUDENT. When you find good mentors, be a good listener and act on their advice and suggestions. I think the best mentors lead by example to help you accomplish your goals, think bigger, and even take on greater goals that you once thought were unreachable. Mentors are not there to solve your problems; it's up to you using their advice and wisdom to help you make informed decisions. All mentor-mentee relationships are different, but in general, mentors are there to hold you accountable, push you to do your very best, and inspire you toward being who you want to be.

Someday you may become a mentor yourself. Think of all the positive points and qualities of your best mentors. A great listener? A person who took time to learn about you and goals? Accessibility? Guidance offered in a positive, productive manner? Your mentors' best qualities are the ones you'll want to emulate.

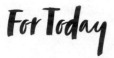

TODAY'S QUOTE

I've had mentors who were kind of the troubadour singer-songwriters, like Merle Haggard, Loretta Lynn, Joni Mitchell, Bob Dylan, and Neil Young, and that's just what I've always liked—people who would talk real honestly about their lives and their circumstances.
—JEWEL

TODAY'S AFFIRMATION

_____

_____

_____

First, identify potential mentors. List the people you know or could get access to who would make good mentors.

What qualities or experience do they have that might make them a good mentor for you?

Which ones are most likely to support and encourage you?

Approach one of the people on your list and ask him or her to mentor you. Again, be sure to define the relationship: Why are you looking for a mentor? What are your goals and how can a mentor help? How will you communicate with each other? How often? What sort of information, guidance, and resources will you need? Assure your potential mentor that you won't be a nuisance, but are really committed to a good mentor-mentee relationship.

Second, prepare for your first meeting with your mentor.

Here are some questions to ask your mentor and get the ball rolling:

What do you wish you knew at my stage of life?
If you could do it all again, what would you do differently?
What have been your most rewarding accomplishments?
What could I be doing better?
What would you do if you were in my situation, at my stage of life, and with my goals?
When did you realize you were on the right path for yourself?

Today's Mental Goal:

_____

Today's Personal Goal:

_____

Today's Spiritual Goal:

_____

MY BADASS REFLECTIONS FOR TODAY

What are you most grateful for today?

Mentally: _____

Physically: _____

Spiritually: _____

What was the biggest success for you today?

Mentally: _____

Physically: _____

Spiritually: _____

What was the biggest challenge for you today? How did you overcome it?

Mentally: _____

Physically: _____

Spiritually: _____

What can you do tomorrow to make it a better day?

Mentally: _____

Physically: _____

Spiritually: _____

CHECKLIST

☐   I completed my habit change challenges.

☐   I made healthy choices today for my mind, body, and spirit.

☐   I've expressed my gratitude for today and all it brings, good and bad.

☐   I've prepared for tomorrow and all the unknowns it might bring.

Day 20
BANISH STRESS

WHEN YOUR HEART pounds because of a rude cashier, a poorly run meeting, or a heated argument with your spouse, that's stress. The cashier, the meeting, and the argument are the stressors.

Although stress can involve happy events (such as getting married, buying a house, getting a promotion, having kids, winning the lottery), we tend to think of stress as coming from sudden overwhelming catastrophic events such as losing a job, getting divorced, or having an accident. Such events are acute stressors. They occur suddenly or have a limited time span, and eventually life calms down. Our nervous system is actually designed to handle acute stresses quite well.

Chronic stress, on the other hand, can wear us down and make us sick, and even has the potential to kill us. Chronic stressors are constant stressors; they include a job you hate, illness, lack of sleep, prolonged financial hardship, or the burden of an abusive relationship. Because chronic stressors occur continuously, our bodies never fully relax, and the result can be illnesses such as depression, anxiety, digestive problems, heart disease, ulcers, fatigue, and skin rashes, among others. About 85 percent of medical problems are stress related.

We all need ways to relieve this stress or we'll end up running on empty and not accomplishing what we want. Try the badass strategies starting on page 170.

Test Your Stress Level

How stressed are you? In a now-famous study published in the *Journal of Psychosomatic Research* in 1964, Dr. Thomas H. Holmes and Dr. Richard H. Rahe created the following do-it-yourself stress test, which has been used and published extensively by many organizations. The test measures Life Change Units (LCUs), from the death of a spouse to getting a traffic ticket. By adding up your LCUs, you can predict the likelihood of coming down with a stress-related illness or accident. Circle the events that have occurred in your life over the past year and add up the LCUs, that correspond with each one.

Death of spouse 100

Divorce 73

Marital separation 65

Detention in jail 63

Death of a close family member 63

Major personal injury or illness 53

Marriage 50

Fired from job 47

Marital reconciliation 45

Retirement 45

Major change in health of a family member 44

Pregnancy 40

Sex difficulties 40

Gaining new family member through birth, adoption, or remarriage 39

Major business readjustment 39

Major change in financial state 38

Death of a close friend 37

Change to different line of work 36

Major increase in the number of arguments with spouse 35

Mortgage/loan for a major purchase (such as a home) 31

Foreclosure of mortgage or loan 30

Major change in responsibilities at work ...29

Son or daughter leaving home 29

Trouble with in-laws 29

Outstanding personal achievement 28

Spouse begins or stops work 26

Begin or end school 26

Change in living conditions (rebuilding, remodeling) 25

Revision of personal habits 24

Trouble with boss 23

Major change in work hours or conditions 20

Change in residence 20

Change in schools 20

Major change in usual type or amount of recreation 19

Major change in church activities 19

Major change in social activities 19

Making a purchase (such as a car) 17

Major change in sleeping habits 16

Major change in number of family get-togethers 15

Major change in eating habits 15

Vacation 13

Christmas or holidays 12

Minor violations of the law 11

RESULTS
Total LCUs below 150: Your chance of an illness or accident within two years is 35 percent.

150 to 300 LCUs: Your chance of an illness or accident within two years is 51 percent.

More than 300 LCUs: Your chance of an illness or accident is 80 percent.

Source: R. H. Rahe et al. 1964. Social stress and illness onset. *Journal of Psychosomatic Research* 8(1): 35–44.

Move Your Body

This is the best stress buster I know. Exercising churns out feel-good endorphins that neutralize stress, along the way making you feel better physically and emotionally. Another physical activity that can mediate stress eating is yoga, one of my favorite practices. It's known to lower stress so that you aren't always engaging in negative behaviors for relief. Yoga has a world of other benefits, too, such as strength, flexibility, and antiaging.

Breathe and Relax

When you're stressed, your sympathetic nervous system (which accelerates your heart rate, constricts your blood vessels, and raises your blood pressure) goes on high alert. If this situation continues without a break, you can feel pretty crappy in no time: fatigue, headaches, muscle tension, irritability, light-headedness, shortness of breath, sleep problems, and stomachaches.

What you need to do is relax using specific relaxation techniques. They can change how you feel, physically and mentally, plus counter the effects of long-term stress.

There are many relaxation techniques, but I find the simplest one is conscious breathing. It's easy to do and will take the edge off and quiet your nerves in no time, and you can do it anytime, anywhere. Here's how:

Lie on your back on an exercise mat or other soft surface. Over a count of three, slowly breathe in through your nose. Count to three again as you exhale through your mouth. Make sure your abdomen expands and contracts easily with each breath. With regular practice, you can discreetly use this technique any time stress hits.

Eat Right, Stress Less

When deficient in certain nutrients, you'll feel anxious, even depressed, because food does affect mood. Low levels of vitamin B12 (available from meats) and B9 or folate (from leafy green vegetables and legumes) have been linked to depression, for example.

Fats such as those found in nuts, seeds, nut butters, and oils like olive oil are stress busters. They make you happy, too—they're a terrific mood lifter. They also tell your body when you're full and prevent you from overeating.

From protein-rich foods, you get amino acids, which the body uses to manufacture the *mood neurotransmitters* dopamine, epinephrine, and norepinephrine. These important brain chemicals help energize you, boost alertness, and enhance concentration. Carbohydrates are broken down to supply blood sugar, or glucose, which triggers the release of insulin into your bloodstream. Insulin promotes the action of tryptophan, an amino acid converted by the brain into the feel-good neurotransmitter serotonin. The best carbs are of course those found in whole grains, fruits, and vegetables because they are slower to be digested and provide nutrients. Combining proteins with these kinds of carbs also slows digestion and keeps blood sugar—and moods—stable.

Other nutrients important for fighting stress and boosting mood are vitamin C (available from citrus fruits and brightly colored fruits and vegetables) and minerals such as zinc (abundant in fish, soybeans, spinach, and egg yolks), magnesium (supplied by whole grains, nuts, fish, and green vegetables), and selenium (plentiful in whole grains, meats, and fish).

Enjoy these foods on a regular basis, too. This means having your meals and snacks at fairly fixed times. Doing so can help you break the habit of impulse eating. Don't skip meals to save calories, either. This can lead to hunger later in the day, and the temptation to overeat.

Healthy snacking will keep you on the straight and narrow, too. I snack a lot through the day. A few of my absolute favorites are:

- 2 hard-boiled eggs + a dollop of peanut butter + a squeeze of applesauce (no sugar added!)
- 1 single-serve guacamole pack + strips of bell peppers + 2 slices of deli meat
- FITAID Fuel Pouch—literally just slurp and go.

...

Sleep Away Stress

While lots of fun things happen in your bed, bad things happen, too, like lack of sleep. Most of us think going to sleep is no big deal. You just go to the bathroom, take off your clothes, put on your jammies, hit the sack, close your eyes, and drift off to the Land of Nod until the next morning. But this is not a true scenario for the estimated fifty to seventy million Americans who log less than six hours of sleep most nights.

You see, when you don't sleep well, very little healing takes place. Energy is not restored, nor are muscles repaired adequately. Important hormones released during sleep are not produced. The next day your brain will have trouble processing thoughts, and you'll feel mentally sluggish.

Lack of sleep makes you more prone to stress. A slew of research has shown that losing sleep makes you crave high-calorie foods. Why? Being sleep-deprived jacks up levels of the stress hormone cortisol and the feed-me hormone ghrelin; production of blood-sugar-controlling insulin gets screwed up, too. The net result is that your body can shift into a weight-gaining mode, and you're stuck in a hunger-craving loop.

Also, a lack of sleep activates the system in the body that controls reward, called the endocannabinoid system. It's the same system that's triggered by marijuana, and when it's activated, it makes people hungrier. Sleep deprivation basically gives you the "munchies," just as marijuana does. You feel hungrier, even though you don't need more food energy than a person getting enough sleep. All of these factors create stress—so you've got to get your shut-eye. It's a stress reliever.

You can fix sleep problems without resorting to sleeping pills. For example:

STOP TWEETING, TEXTING, EMAILING, and so forth at least an hour prior to bedtime. Your computers, smartphones, and tablets emit blue light, which disrupts the activity of melatonin, the sleep hormone.

WATCH WHAT YOU DRINK AT NIGHT. Coffee, unless it's decaf, will keep you up. So will too much alcohol. Booze depresses the central nervous system, and as it wears off, the system rebounds—which can make you wakeful in the middle of the night and have less deep sleep.

GRAB A HEAVIER BLANKET. The added weight of the blanket makes us feel more "tucked in," "hugged," and ultimately safer—all of which translates into fewer restless nights.

WORRY NOT. A lot of people sleep badly because they take the day's problems home with them. They're counting their problems instead of sheep (which I don't recommend that you to do, either, because watching imaginary flocks flinging themselves over fences actually makes it harder to drift off, scientists have found!).

USE FOOD. It's not surprising that food can fix poor sleep. After all, sleep recharges the energy we get from food, and among other things, helps rid the body of harmful chemicals. Sleep also enhances the power of disease-fighting nutrients called antioxidants. Two proven foods to eat prior to bedtime are bananas and yogurt. Bananas are rich in three important minerals: magnesium, potassium, and calcium. All three nutrients together act as muscle relaxers and are known to be effective in treating insomnia. Plus, bananas contain the sleep-inducing amino acid tryptophan, which ultimately turns into serotonin and melatonin in the brain. Yogurt contains a rich supply of two natural sleep aids: tryptophan and calcium. Calcium plays a direct role in the production of melatonin.

SIP TEA. Can't get your eyes to shut when your head hits the pillow? Sip some valerian tea. It contains natural sedative compounds that may reduce the time it takes for you to fall asleep. One of the oldest and most widely used herbal remedies in the world, chamomile acts as a mild sedative and slumber inducer.

Change Your Response

It's not the stressor that gets you riled up—it's your reaction to it. So an effective coping strategy is to understand when you have the leverage to change things and when you don't. When something is clearly beyond your control (such as another person's behavior), you can either try to avoid the stressful situation or person or work to change your reaction to it.

Let's go back to the rude cashier or the argumentative spouse for a moment. If someone lashes out at you, respond calmly, and if it helps, think of the rude comment or argument as a package you can return unopened. Don't take things personally.

Control your vibe, too. People often mirror the behaviors of others. So if you listen, have empathy, and smile, they're more likely to act the same way toward you.

You might have to rearrange your life to tackle stress. Many people bring stress upon themselves by refusing to say no and overextending themselves, so be a badass and set realistic goals. Put more balance in your life so that you have time for pleasure, relaxation, and spiritual fulfillment—all life choices that will counteract the negative effects of stress.

For Today

TODAY'S QUOTE

The greatest weapon against stress is our ability to choose one thought over another.
—WILLIAM JAMES

TODAY'S AFFIRMATION

_____

_____

_____

Create a personal stress management plan. Here's how:

Step 1. Identify your stress triggers. What really stresses you out? Finances? Family members? Certain people? Work pressures?

Step 2. Develop coping strategies. These include exercising, relaxation and meditation, better nutrition, and improved sleep quality. Which ones will you commit to?

Step 3. Implement stress management tools. Remember, you can either change the situation that causes stress or change your reaction to it, or both. When deciding which option to choose, consider the following:

I will identify and accept the things I can't change. Don't try to control the uncontrollable (which is most things in life!). Acknowledging that certain things are beyond your dominion is a tremendous stress reliever. You can only control and change yourself.

I will avoid unnecessary stress. This could mean saying no more often, staying away from stressful people, making a household budget, or finding another route to avoid traffic jams.

I will change the situation. You might manage your time better, learn to speak up more, or be willing to compromise—whatever it takes to constructively avoid the problem or issue in the future.

I will alter my response. If you can't change the source of your stress, change your reaction to it. Ask yourself: Will this issue matter a month or a year from now? Change your emotional responses to stress with realistic, positive, and constructive self-talk. For example, instead of thinking that a situation is horrible or catastrophic or the "worst thing ever," tell yourself: *Things are never as bad as I can make them seem.* This defuses your stress response.

Today's Mental Goal:

_____

Today's Personal Goal:

_____

Today's Spiritual Goal:

_____

MY BADASS REFLECTIONS FOR TODAY

What are you most grateful for today?

Mentally: _____

Physically: _____

Spiritually: _____

What was the biggest success for you today?

Mentally: _____

Physically: _____

Spiritually: _____

What was the biggest challenge for you today? How did you overcome it?

Mentally: _____

Physically: _____

Spiritually: _____

What can you do tomorrow to make it a better day?

Mentally: _____

Physically: _____

Spiritually: _____

CHECKLIST

☐   I completed my habit change challenges.

☐   I made healthy choices today for my mind, body, and spirit.

☐   I've expressed my gratitude for today and all it brings, good and bad.

☐   I've prepared for tomorrow and all the unknowns it might bring.

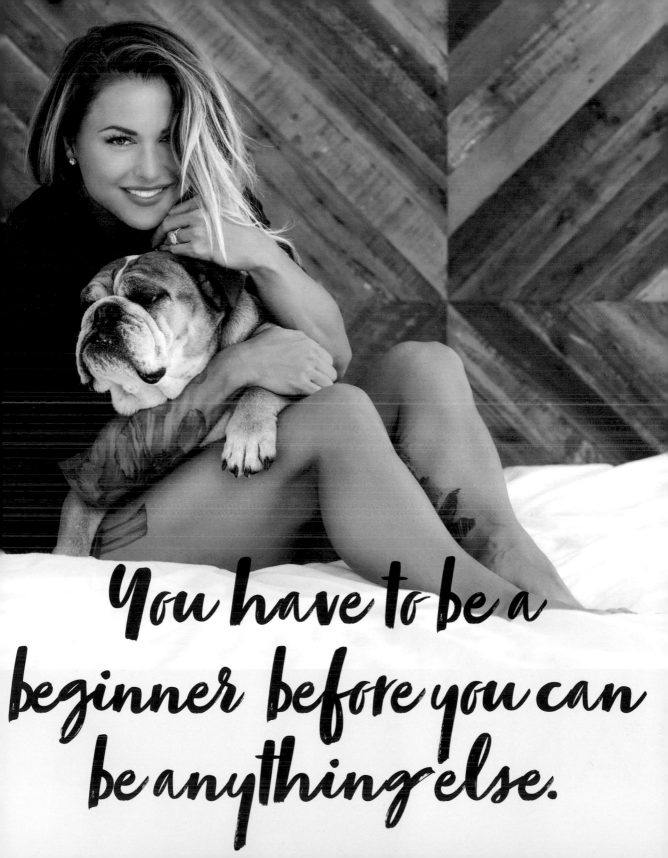

You have to be a beginner before you can be anything else.

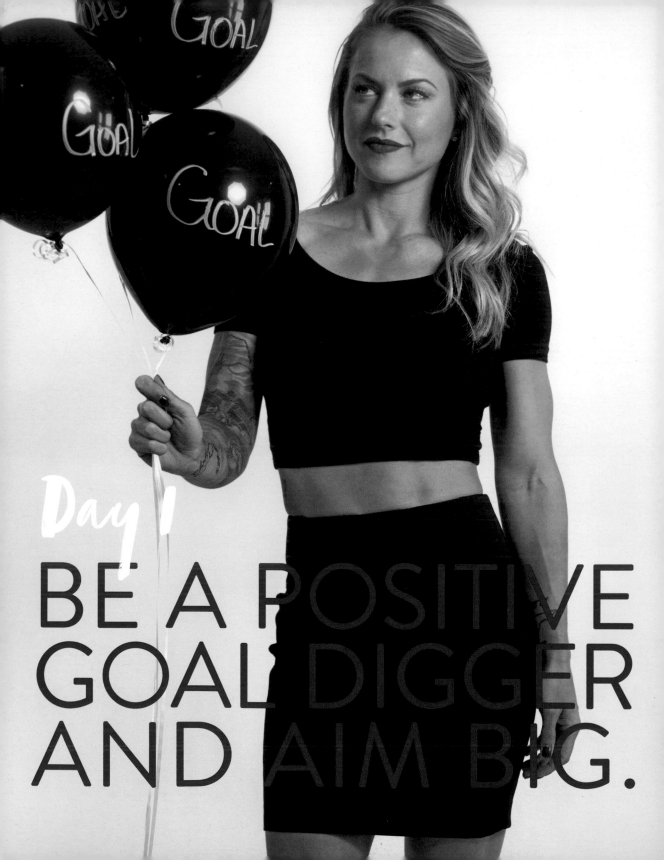

Day 1

BE A POSITIVE
GOAL DIGGER
AND AIM BIG.

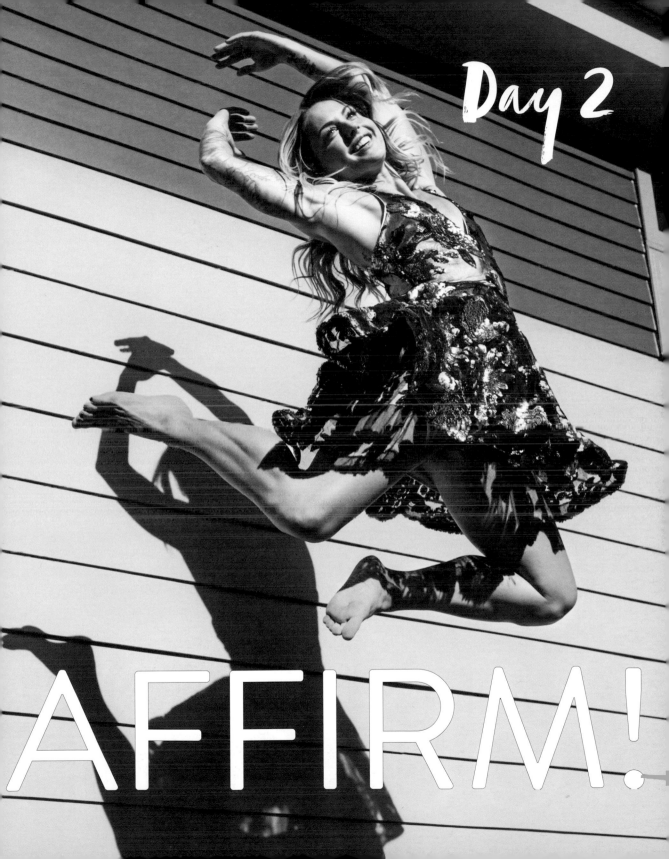

Day 2

AFFIRM!

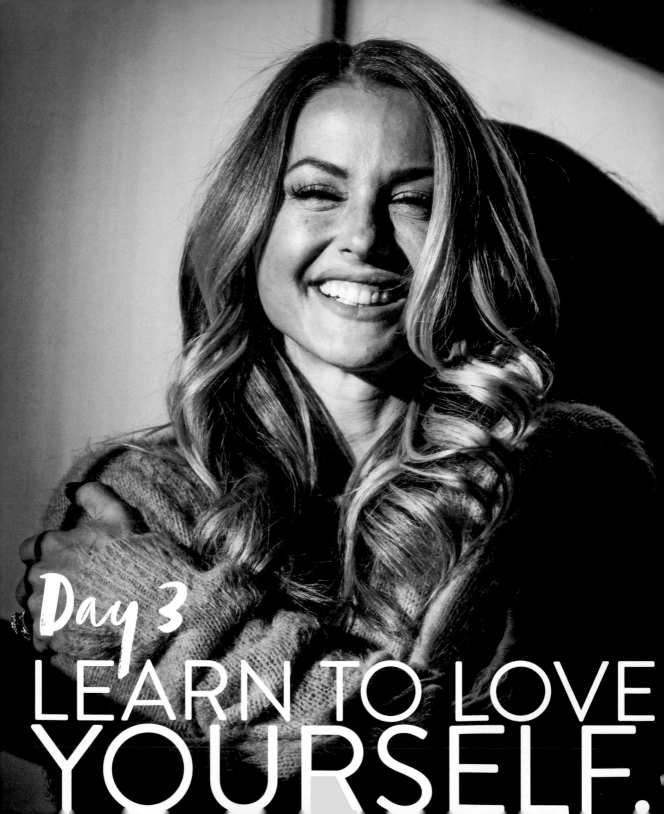

Day 3
LEARN TO LOVE
YOURSELF.

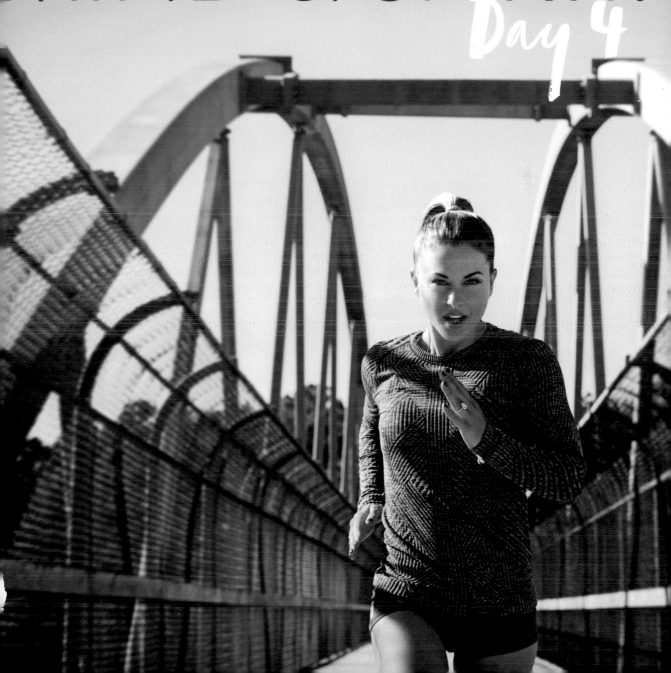

EXERCISE YOUR MIND & SPIRIT.
Day 4

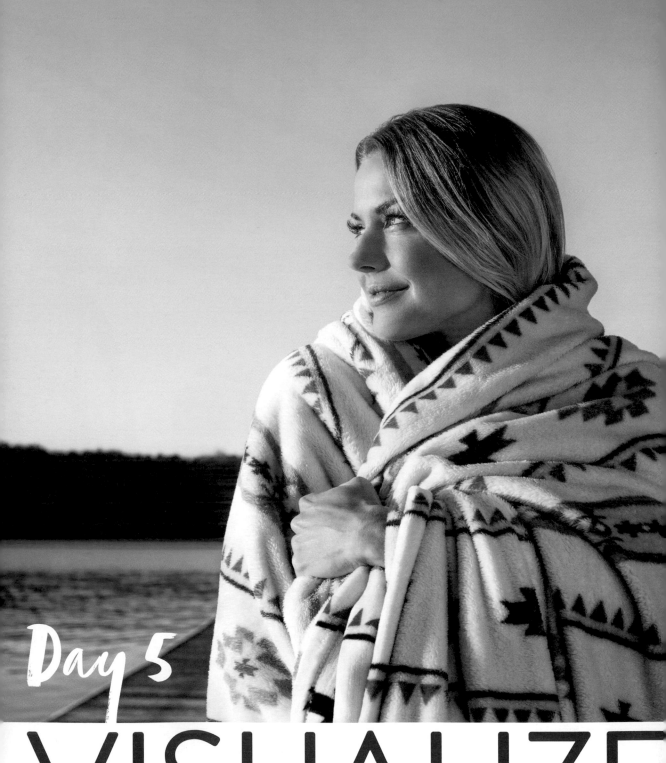

Day 5

VISUALIZE

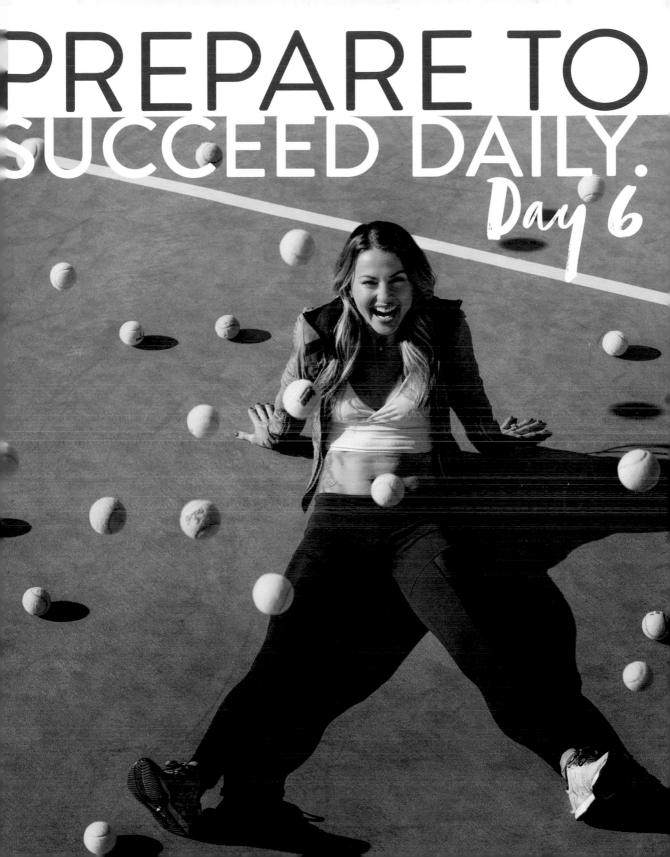

PREPARE TO SUCCEED DAILY.

Day 6

Day 7
BE A RELENTLESS
REBEL.

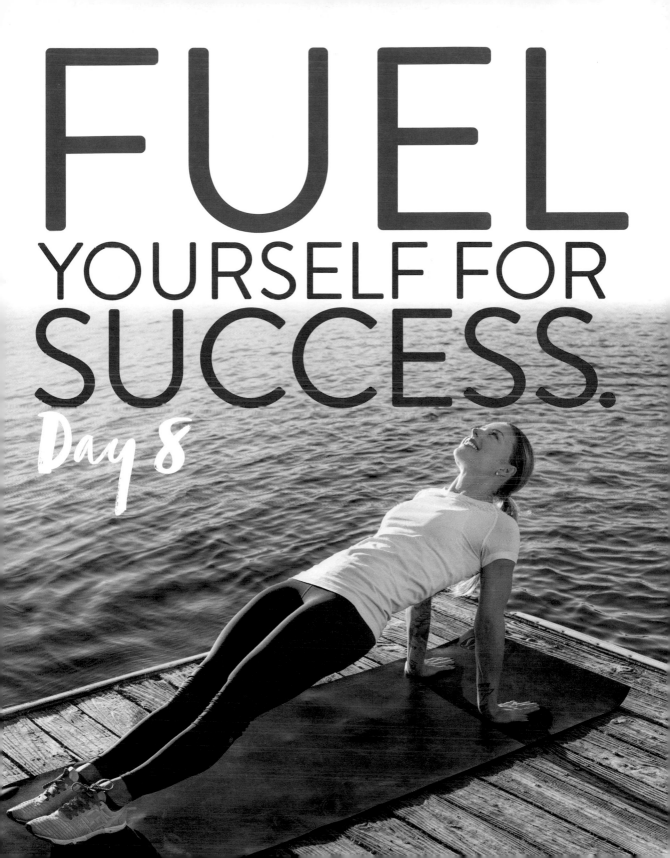

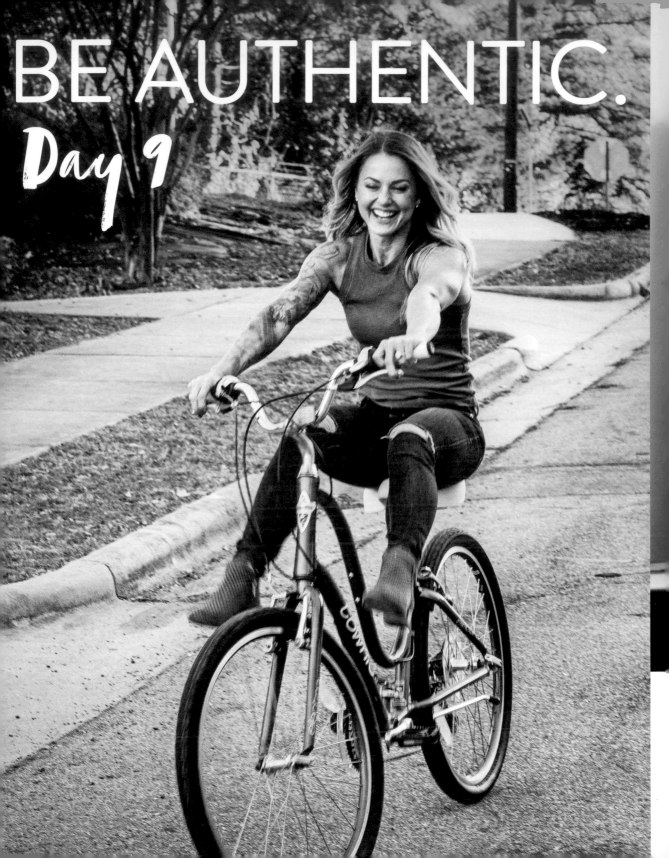

BE AUTHENTIC.

Day 9

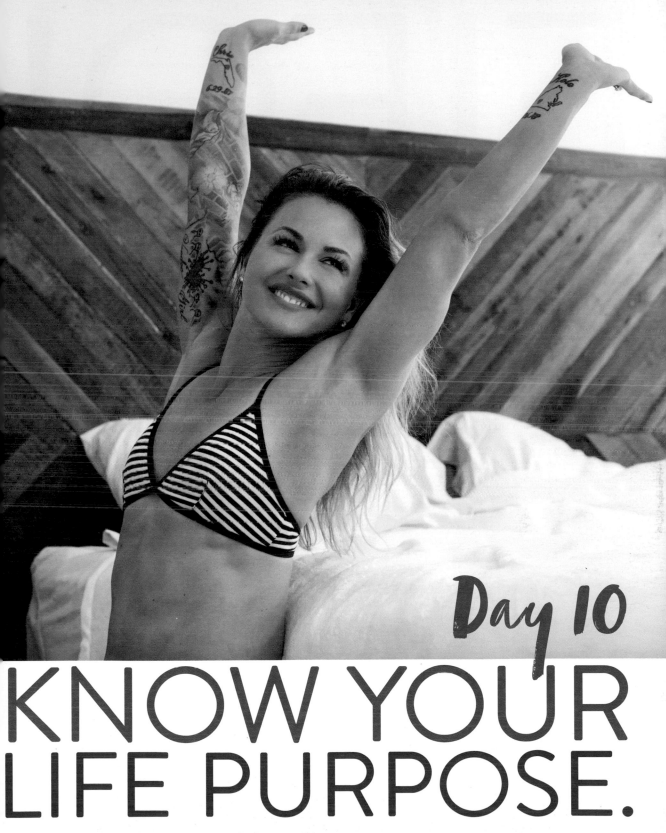

Day 10

KNOW YOUR LIFE PURPOSE.

FIFO!
Day II

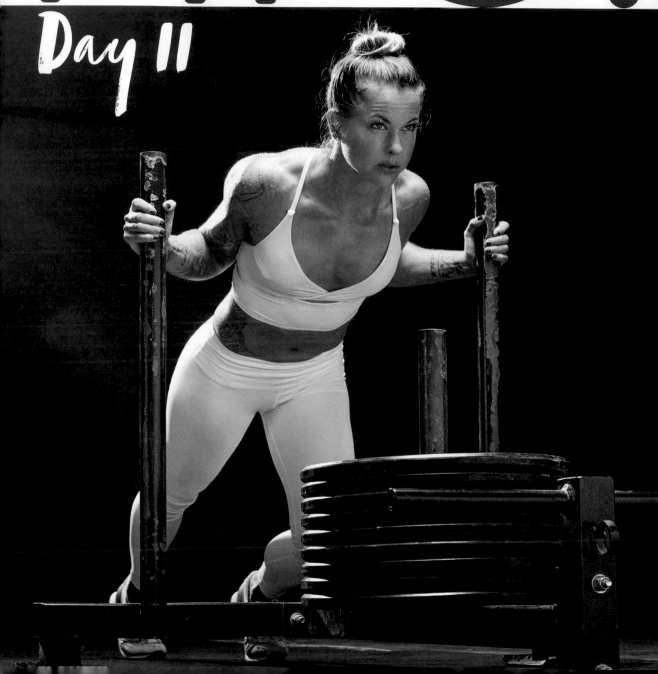

Day 12

DESCRIBE YOUR
LEGACY.

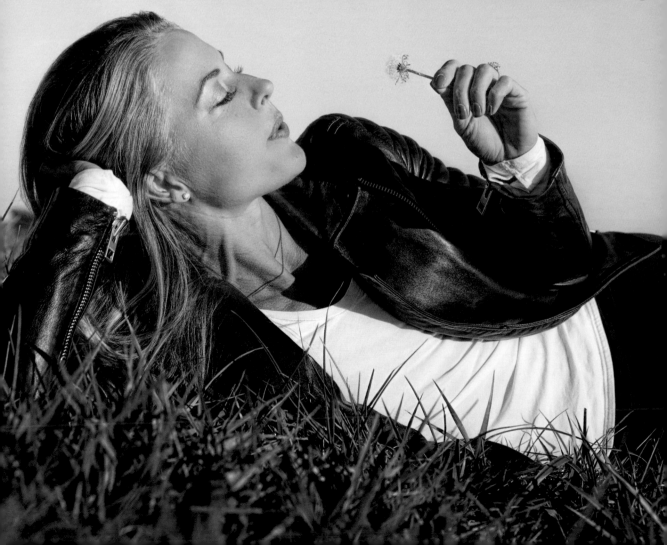

Day 13
LAYER IN CHANGE.

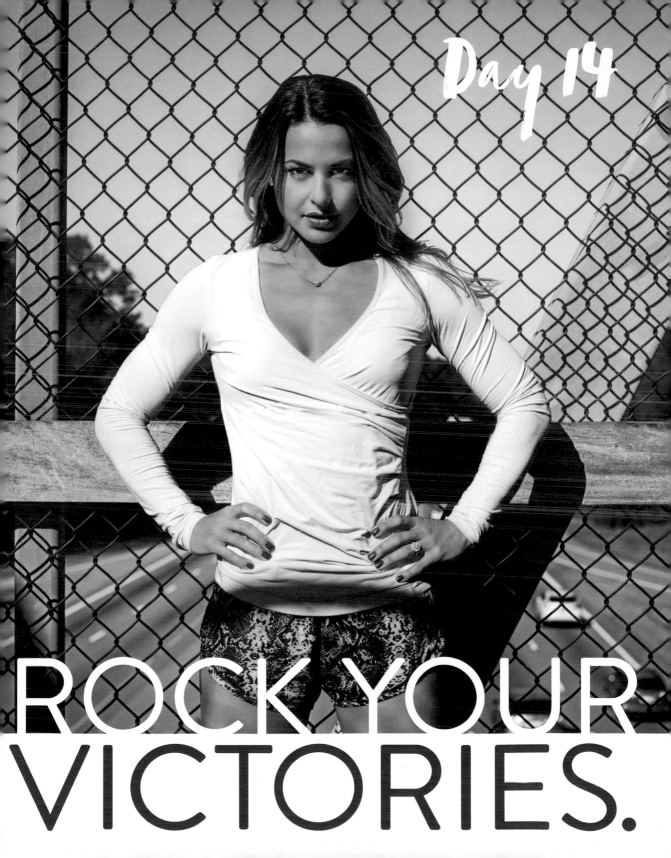

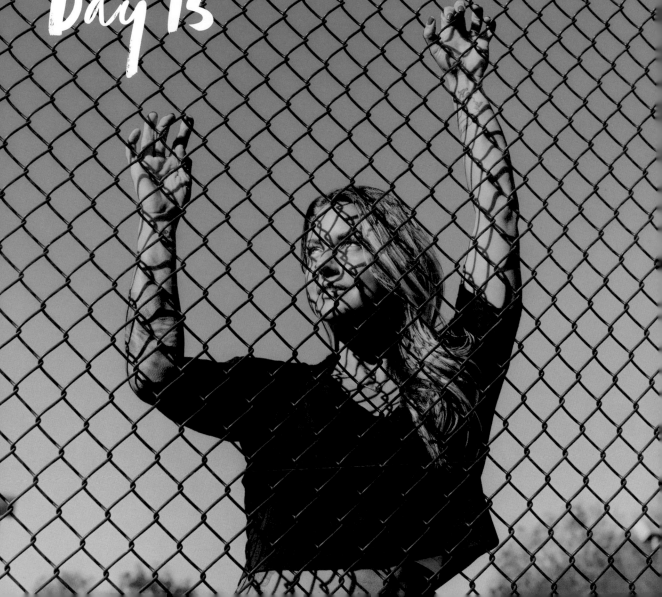

ELIMINATE EXCUSES.

Day 15

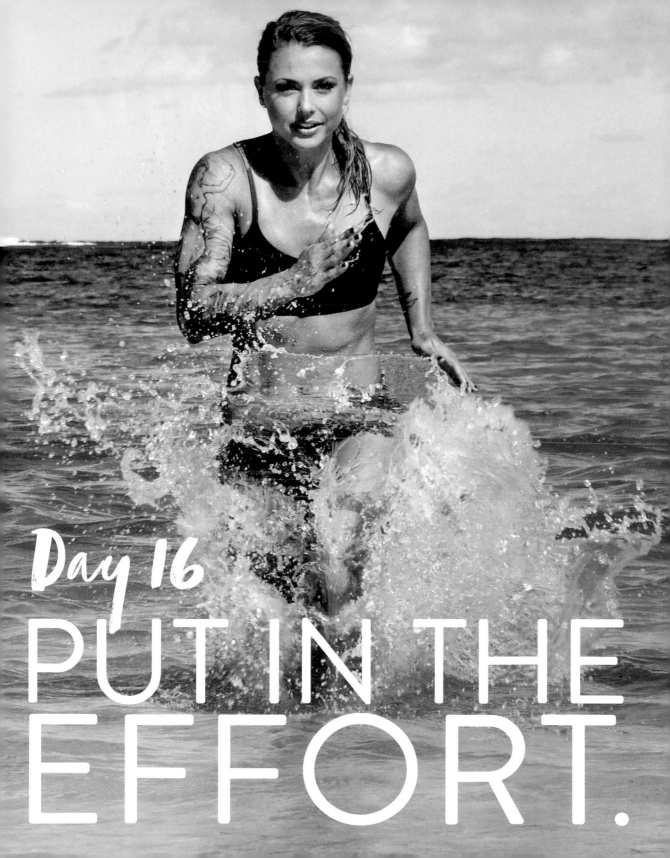

Day 16
PUT IN THE
EFFORT.

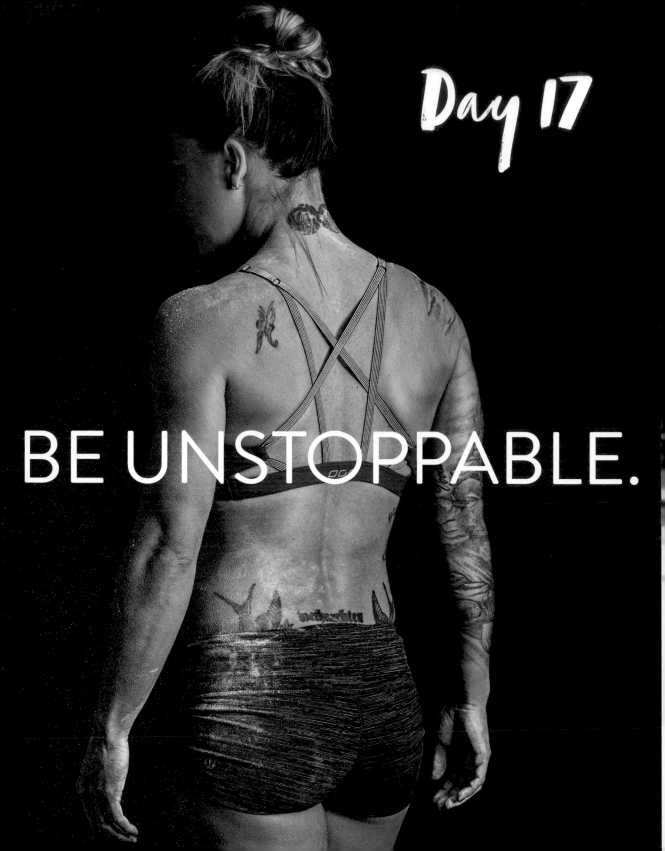

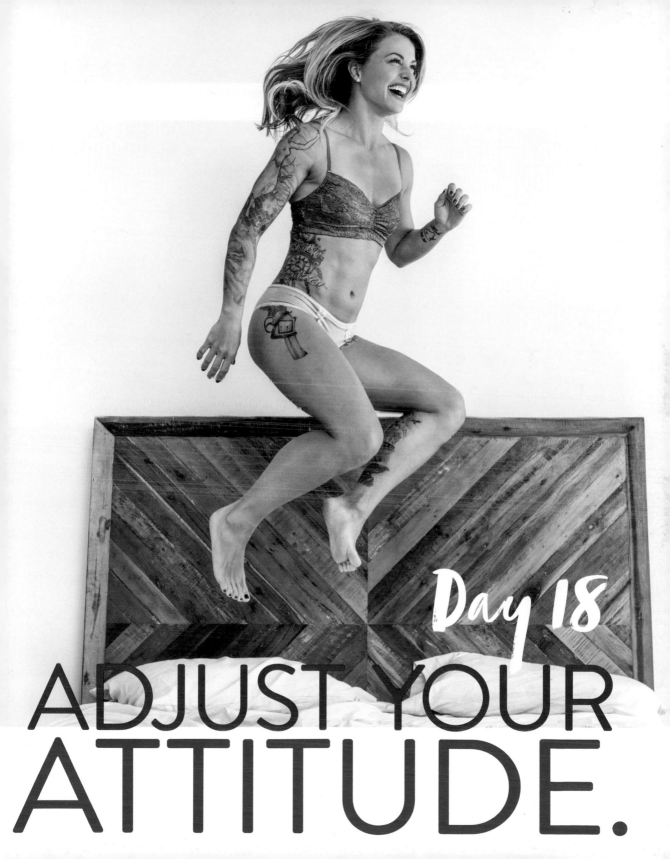

Day 18

ADJUST YOUR
ATTITUDE.

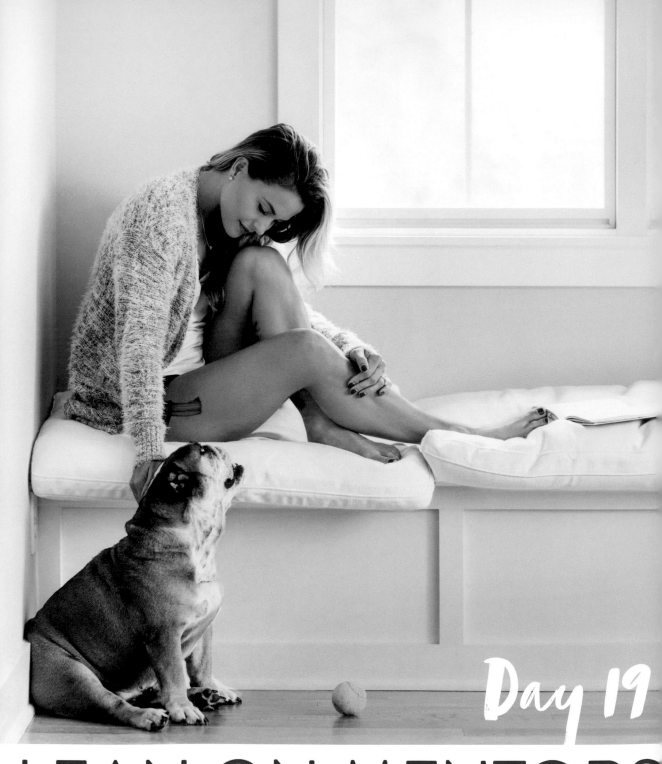

Day 19

LEAN ON MENTORS

BANISH STRESS.

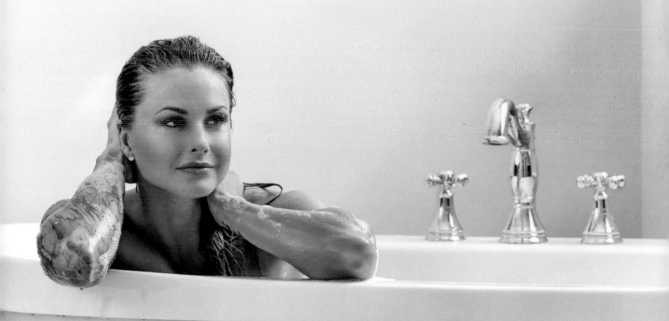

Day 20

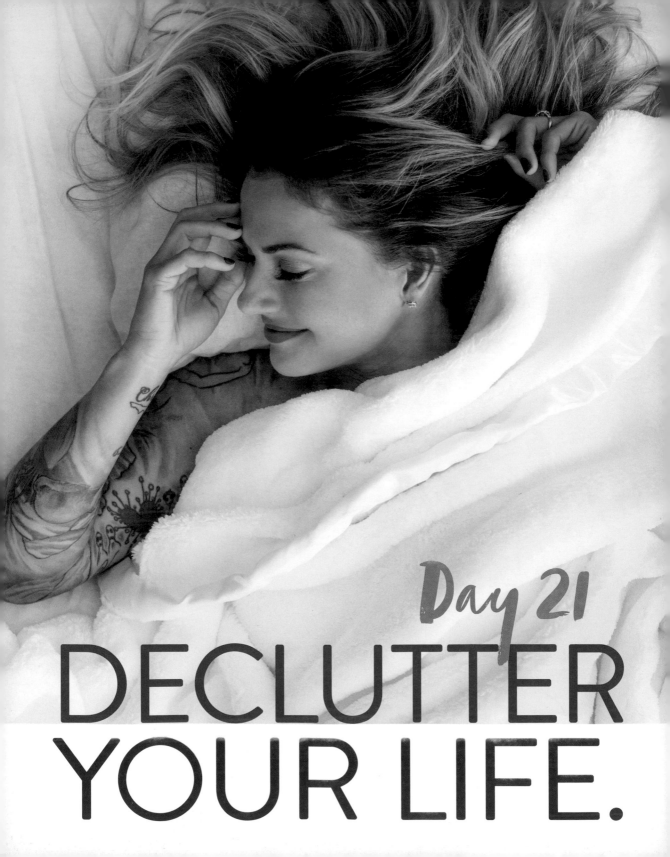

Day 21

DECLUTTER
YOUR LIFE.

CHANGE
THE SCENERY.

Day 22

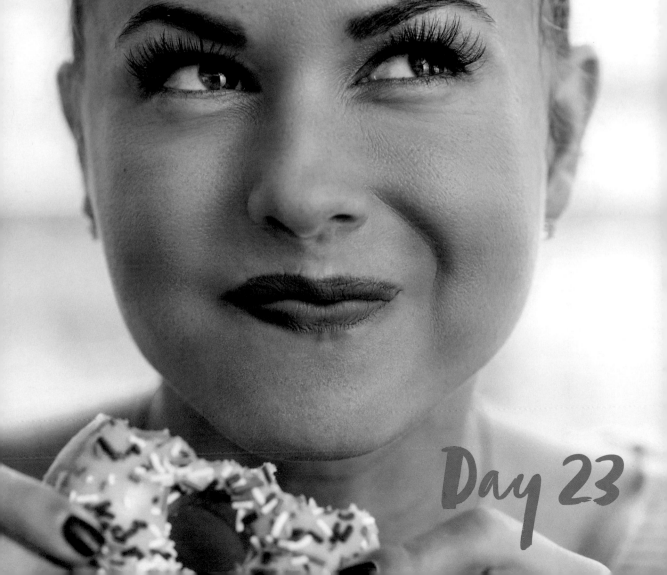

DON'T FORGET THE CHOCOLATE: MODERATION AND SELF-CONTROL.

Day 23

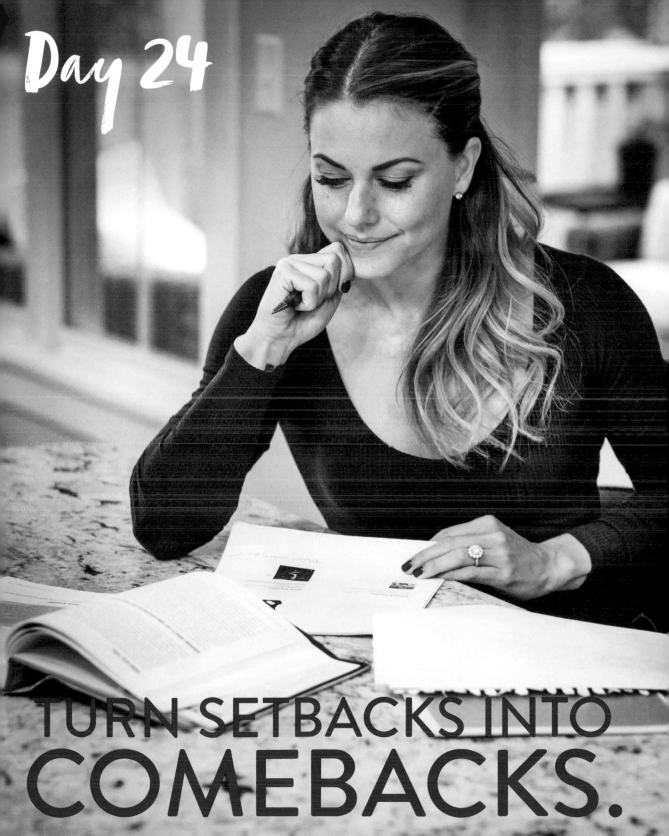

Day 24

TURN SETBACKS INTO
COMEBACKS.

TRAIN YOUR BRAIN.

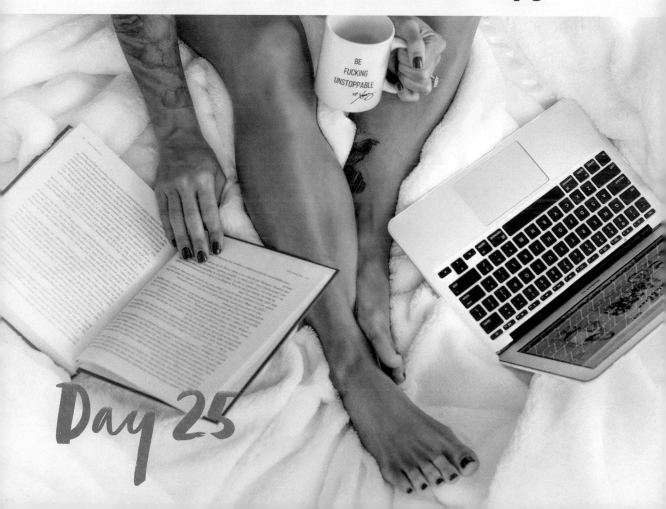

Day 25

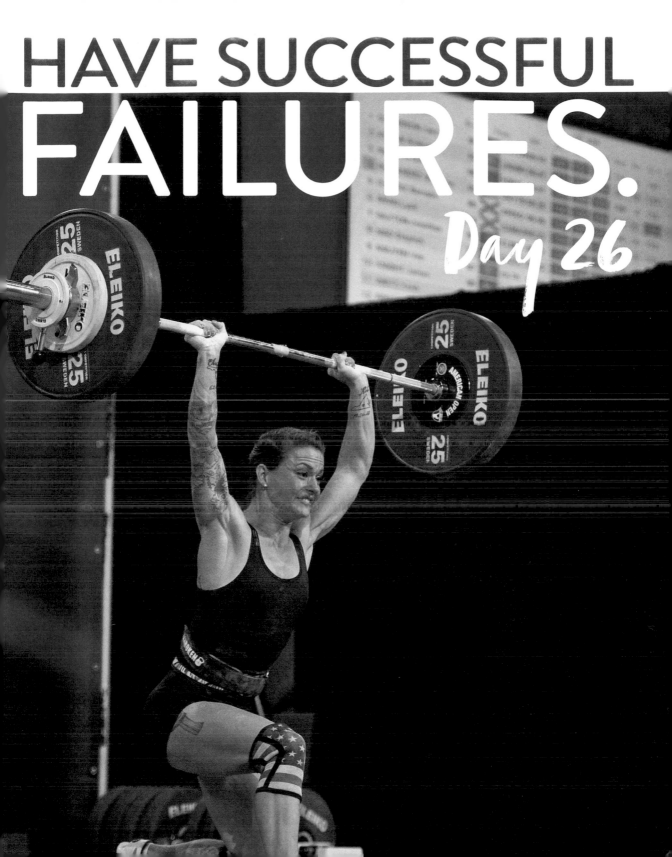

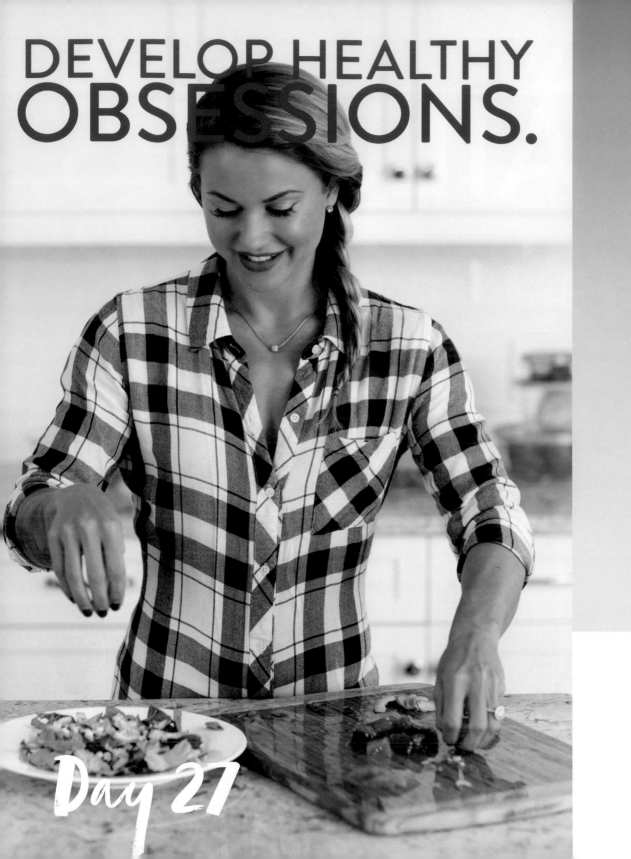

DEVELOP HEALTHY OBSESSIONS.

Day 27

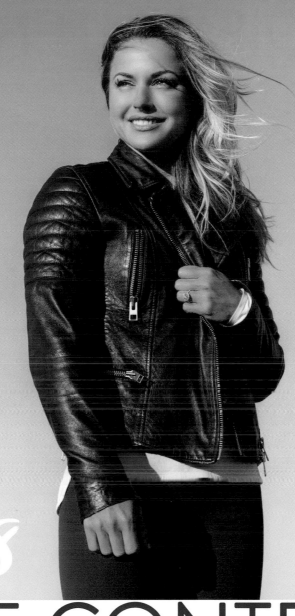

Day 28

TAKE CONTROL
OF ROLLERCOASTER
EMOTIONS.

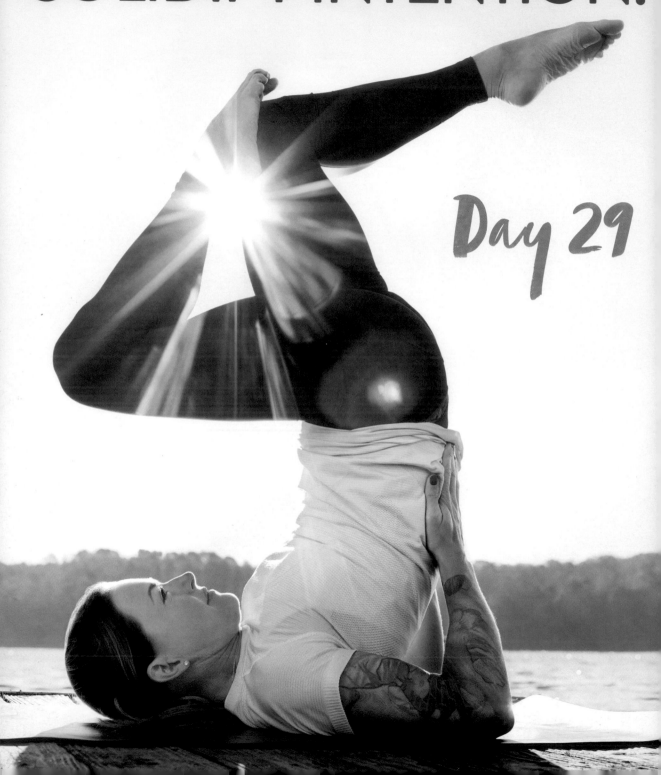

SOLIDIFY INTENTION.

Day 29

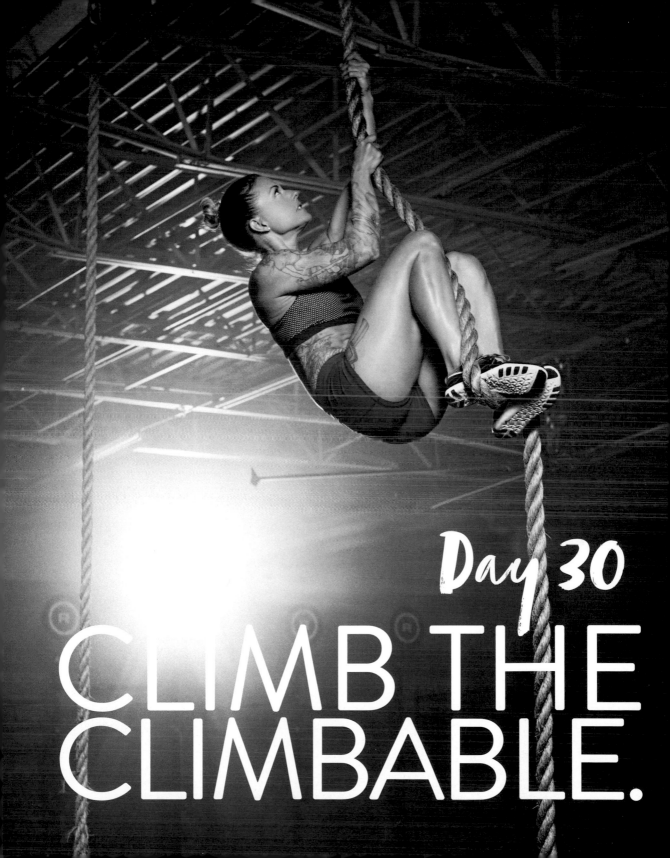

Day 30

CLIMB THE CLIMBABLE.

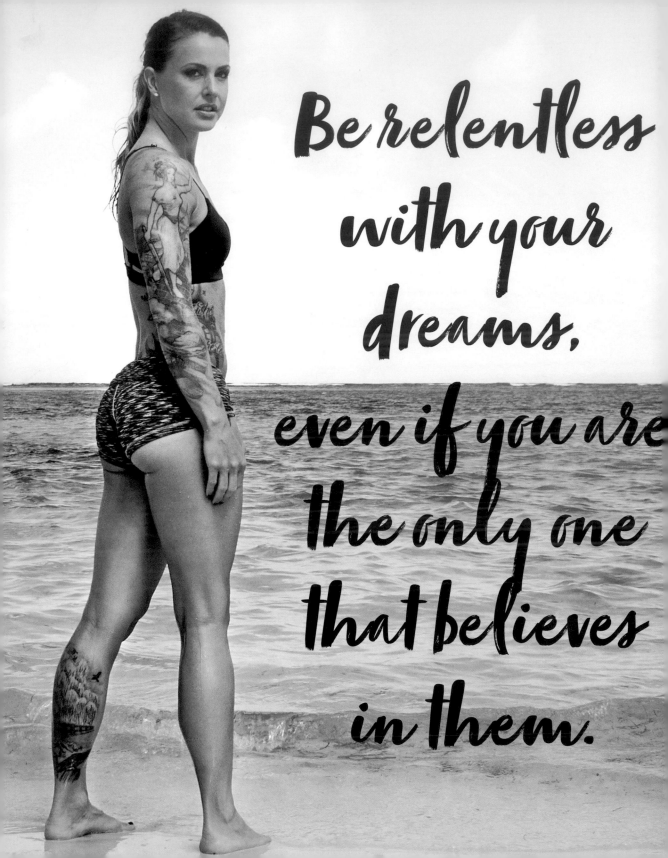

Be relentless with your dreams, even if you are the only one that believes in them.

Day 21

DECLUTTER YOUR LIFE

LATELY I'VE STARTED becoming selfish with my space. *Selfish* may not be the right word to use here; perhaps *protective* would be better. I know what's important to my happiness and what is stressing me out. Often the stressor is the unimportant stuff—you know, plain old clutter.

Living or working in a cluttered space has the potential to stress you out and even make you physically ill. Research has shown that women who were asked to do tasks in cluttered environments had far higher levels of the stress hormone cortisol than when they performed the same task in tidy surroundings. Elevated cortisol increases your risk of cardiovascular disease, insomnia, weight gain, and anxiety. Clutter is bad for your health!

For today, start decluttering your life. Take a look at what surrounds you; if it doesn't bring you happiness, now is the perfect time to let it go. Learning to say no to some things in order to say yes to what's important to you takes practice, but it's a huge step in the right direction—toward acknowledging that your needs and your health matter.

How do you begin? Where do you begin?

START SMALL. Clutter can be so overwhelming that you don't even want to tackle it. This is because even though you get stressed out by the clutter around you, for many of us, any attempt to reduce the clutter causes even more stress. To get around this vicious circle, devote a few minutes daily to a little decluttering, like cleaning out the utensil drawer in your kitchen or clearing off horizontal surfaces, rather than one unachievable ambition, such as decluttering your whole house. Just seeing a cleared-off kitchen counter, dresser, or desktop will motivate you to do more. You might think a few minutes a day will barely put a dent in the monumental mess, but it's a start.

PROGRESS FROM SMALL SPACES TO A ROOM AT A TIME. Set up a decluttering schedule by which you tidy up one room a day or one room a week. For example:

- The kitchen. Pantries and shelves can get pretty icky with spilled spices, dripping condiment bottles, spilled flour, and junk food that shouldn't be there in the first place. Restore order by removing everything and wiping off the shelves. Toss out expired items and junk food, and then begin restocking. In my pantry, I like to categorize and sort items: nuts and oatmeal on one shelf; rice, noodles, and other things on other shelves.

  In my fridge and freezer, I keep items superorganized. I use glass containers instead of plastic, but fall back on zip-top bags when I need to. I use both of these to prepare and package individual serving sizes for my food. I place my carb servings on the top shelf of my fridge, the protein servings on the middle shelf, and the rest of my food in the lower compartments. I organize my frozen food in the same way. This level of organization may not be for you, but it can help make life less complicated and saves lots of time in the long run. Give it a try! You'll be surprised at how it eases your food prep and destresses your life.

- The bathroom. Sponges, facecloths, and cosmetics can be organized in utensil organizers (like those you use in your kitchen) placed in drawers. I like clutter-free horizontal surfaces, so I place most items out of sight but easily reachable.

- Closets. Although a lot of us have limited closet space, there's nothing more frustrating and overwhelming than crammed closets that spill stuff when you open them. It's always hard to find anything and can be quite stressful. The best organizing principle for me is to organize by item—pants, jeans, and skirts on one rung; blouses and dresses on another; and sweaters, T-shirts, and workout clothes on shelves. I color-code each rung, too. I keep my shoes in shoe organizers or on designated shelves in my closet. If you haven't worn an item for two years, unless it's a very expensive piece, be ruthless and get rid of it. I like to detox my wardrobe at least twice a year.

- The utility room. Solve laundry problems once and for all with a family laundry sorter. Get everyone to separate out black, white, and colored items. It will clear bedroom floors and you'll zip through laundry day.

- The living room or den. Make nicely ordered bookshelves part of your decor. Try using woven cubbies to store all your magazines, game consoles, DVDs, and even the knitting!

- Big areas. For larger spaces, such as your garage, attic, or basement, carve out a weekend for decluttering and cleanup. Make the task more fun by listening to music, keeping some refreshing drinks on hand, and taking breaks as often as you need them.

DECIDE WHAT TO TOSS. As you go through your house, remember that decluttering is not all about throwing away memories or mementos. It is all about trashing real junk—the stuff that is no longer useful or meaningful.

APPLY THE "ONE IN, ONE OUT" PHILOSOPHY. For every new item you bring into the house, let one go. In other words, for every item that comes into your home, something else should go out in turn.

ORGANIZE AS YOU GO THROUGH YOUR STUFF. Take four boxes and label them TRASH, STORAGE, DONATE, and FOR SALE. Then follow through on the designations.

PRACTICE CLUTTER PREVENTION. Maintain your decluttering momentum! Sort through and throw away unwanted mail and papers the day you receive them. Take ten minutes each weekend to declutter. As for new stuff, ask yourself if you really need it. Set limits on what you bring into your home.

Enjoy the benefits of decluttering. It definitely simplifies your life. You'll be less stressed, happier, and more clearheaded and in control. And you'll actually be able to find things you've misplaced.

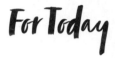

TODAY'S QUOTE

Every minute you spend looking through clutter, wondering where you put this or that, being unable to focus because you're not organized costs you: time you could have spent with family or friends, time you could have been productive around the house, time you could have been making money.
—JEAN CHATZKY

TODAY'S AFFIRMATION

_____

_____

_____

TODAY'S CHALLENGE

Start small. Forget about cleaning your whole house. Select one room of your house, or even one area such as your desk or pantry, and declutter it. Step back and ask yourself how it felt to clean that single area.

If you have more decluttering to do, create a plan to get it done. Maybe you decide to devote just ten minutes a day to decluttering, or you tackle a room a day, or perhaps reserve a few hours each weekend to the task.

Be grateful! Simply focus on how fortunate you are to have a house or residence to clean. This thought will change your attitude toward decluttering in an instant!

Today's Mental Goal:

_____

Today's Personal Goal:

_____

Today's Spiritual Goal:

_____

MY BADASS REFLECTIONS FOR TODAY

What are you most grateful for today?

Mentally: _____

Physically: _____

Spiritually: _____

What was the biggest success for you today?

Mentally: _____

Physically: _____

Spiritually: _____

What was the biggest challenge for you today? How did you overcome it?

Mentally: _____

Physically: _____

Spiritually: _____

What can you do tomorrow to make it a better day?

Mentally: _____

Physically: _____

Spiritually: _____

CHECKLIST

☐ I completed my habit change challenges.

☐ I made healthy choices today for my mind, body, and spirit.

☐ I've expressed my gratitude for today and all it brings, good and bad.

☐ I've prepared for tomorrow and all the unknowns it might bring.

Day 22

CHANGE THE SCENERY

THE ROAR OF powerful engines . . . the fans whooping and hollering . . . the whoosh of the air gun—these were the louder-than-a-rock-concert sounds I'd hear every weekend as a tire changer on a NASCAR pit crew.

Yep, that was my job for a few years, and what an adrenaline rush. I had to be able to comfortably change a tire in split seconds, and I loved it.

How in the world did I land in the dusty, ear-splitting pits? I'm always looking for a new experience to add to my list of adventures, so when a friend suggested in 2012 that I go to a NASCAR recruiting event, I was game.

Dressed in a cute little workout suit and no grease under my prettily painted fingernails, I thought I'd be auditioning to drive a car. No—it would be for changing tires in a pit crew. Uh-oh! Aside from casually watching races with my family back home in Lynchburg, Virginia, I knew nothing about pit stops.

There was a competition to see how fast we could jack a car, hang a tire, and hit the lug nuts. I was able to jack the car, but not very well. Give me a break—it weighs more than 4,000 pounds! I could hang the tire accurately, though, and when it came to hitting the lug nuts, I nailed it. I was the only girl there, and I was able to hit five lug nuts off in 1.7 seconds, beating all the guys there. The NASCAR Sprint Cup had an average hand speed of 1.2 seconds for all five lug nuts to be removed, so even on my first day, I was hitting lug nuts almost as fast as professional pit crewers. Everyone saw me do this, but they were still shocked. They couldn't believe this kind of performance came from me, standing only five foot three and weighing 118 pounds.

I loved it. I felt like I had walked into the middle of something great.

Not long afterward, I got a call from Turner Motorsports offering me a job as a tire changer. I had a full plate at the time—managing my CrossFit gym, coaching classes, teaching bodyweight boot camps, doing seminars every weekend, and training for CrossFit competitions. I was hesitant, but the lure of the track and the brute force of changing tires pulled me in. Eventually I joined the Michael Waltrip Racing team and held the distinction of being the first and only female full-time member of a NASCAR pit crew at the Cup level, the sport's highest level of professional competition.

Working in a pit crew takes a lot of devotion and a lot of hard work. To be superproficient, it's a matter of practice, practice, practice. All week, I'd be doing training drills to build technique and muscle memory. We'd rehearse pit stops so that on race day we'd be as quick, strong, and focused as possible. We'd look at videotapes of our previous performance to see what we could do better. Pit crews are important for NASCAR success. It's possible for a driver to pass several cars, even win the race, because of a quick tire change and fill-up.

I lived and breathed NASCAR during this time of my life. Being a pit crew member meant everything to me, but mostly, I felt like I was a role model. I was showing young women everywhere that anything is possible, especially if you open your mind and heart to trying something new and changing the scenery of your life.

There's always energy buzzing around any new endeavor you take on. That energy is really a form of fear or anxiety. Use it to move forward and "change the scenery" of your life. Whenever I've ventured into new territory, I've worked really hard to use that energy and transform it into excitement and focus for the project to come. That energy is like emotional high-octane fuel to propel me forward and conquer all the what-ifs that could stall me.

So make a habit of saying yes more often, no matter how anxious, frightened, or resistant you might feel at first. You may find that things you didn't believe you could enjoy become some of your new favorite activities.

That's exactly what happened to me when I tried CrossFit and auditioned for NASCAR. Had I not started CrossFit, I would have stayed in bad shape and in a life rut. Had I not gone out for NASCAR, you probably would never have heard of me. Now I know there's no failure—except in not trying.

I get that changing the scenery of your life can seem scary. You might be afraid of what you'll encounter. You might think it's easier to stick with the tried and true. That way you're less likely to fail!

But the truth is, the only way to get out of ruts is to try bold new things. If you don't, you'll never know whether you could have achieved and enjoyed more. Staying in your comfort zone may feel safe, but you risk achieving less than what you're truly capable of.

When considering a new venture, do some research, consult wise mentors, and get a handle on its full scope. Before I committed to NASCAR, I researched pit crew development and anything else I could find about it. I became obsessed with learning more. I did the research, I became knowledgeable, and I went for it when the time was right.

Make sure your heart is in it, too. Let's say you want to do something in the fitness arena. Find an activity that sparks your interest: ice skating, salsa dancing, stand-up paddleboarding. Or if you feel the urge to change jobs, think about professions you've always been interested in but never pursued. Same thing goes for physical scenery. Maybe you've always dreamed of living in the mountains, by the shore, or out west. If you have the means and the flexibility, look into it and see what it takes. Then go for it!

It's all about making yourself number one and thinking about what you want to do with the rest of your life. Ask yourself: Isn't it about time to give your life more meaning and purpose? To finally allow yourself the happiness you want and deserve?

Keep your eyes wide open . . . and be on the lookout for things that interest and excite you. Make a new friend; hang out with someone you haven't before. Investigate resources outside your circle to gain new and different perspectives. Move outside your familiar comfort zone, beginning today.

Do something you've always dreamed of doing: playing a musical instrument, writing a book, or creating artwork.

Get involved in causes you care deeply about—the environment, opportunities for kids, politics, the homeless—or other ways you've wanted to give back.

Start your own business.

Pursue a new hobby, sport, workout, or physical challenge. I remember the first time I ever did a 24-inch box jump. I was only about a year into CrossFit and just a little more out of smoking. The guys I worked out with (this was in Iraq) always said if you can do it one time, you can do it as many as times as you need to. The workout took me more than 45 minutes to complete. But I did all rounds, holding a 20-pound ball and jumping on a 24-inch box. It was a mental breakthrough as well as a huge accomplishment.

Whatever it is, seek to discover anything that makes you feel alive, passionate, and connected to something bigger than yourself. There is no right or wrong; just see what shows up! Too often we focus on seeking a *destination*—something tangible at the end of our journey. Instead, focus on finding a sense of *direction*. Once you identify what sparks your laughter, brings a smile to your face, what evokes passion and pride within you—then and only then are you on your way to reinvention.

If you aren't happy with where you are in life or with the path you see your future leading toward, make a change! Life is way too short to just mosey along through it unhappy with yourself and your accomplishments.

So say yes more often, take risks, and change the scenery. When it works, you win. If it doesn't, you gain wisdom.

Nothing happens for you unless you're willing to try new things. Life is about fun, challenges, resourcefulness, and opportunity. It's the experiences that you'll remember, not the nights of watching TV, binge-watching shows on Netflix, or obsessing over social media.

For Today

TODAY'S QUOTE

Life is like a dogsled team. If you ain't the lead dog,
the scenery never changes.
—LEWIS GRIZZARD

TODAY'S AFFIRMATION

_____

_____

_____

_____

TODAY'S CHALLENGE

Try something new. Start thinking about ways to change your scenery, whether that's moving to a new place, renovating your current one, applying for a more challenging job, or simply trying a new form of exercise. What is something new you'd like to try?

Explore the payoffs. If you changed your scenery, how would you benefit? In the space below or in your journal, write down five benefits of changing your scenery and trying something new:

_____

_____

_____

_____

Today's Mental Goal:

_____

Today's Personal Goal:

_____

Today's Spiritual Goal:

_____

MY BADASS REFLECTIONS FOR TODAY

What are you most grateful for today?

Mentally: _____

Physically: _____

Spiritually: _____

What was the biggest success for you today?

Mentally: _____

Physically: _____

Spiritually: _____

What was the biggest challenge for you today? How did you overcome it?

Mentally: _____

Physically: _____

Spiritually: _____

What can you do tomorrow to make it a better day?

Mentally: _____

Physically: _____

Spiritually: _____

CHECKLIST

☐ I completed my habit change challenges.

☐ I made healthy choices today for my mind, body, and spirit.

☐ I've expressed my gratitude for today and all it brings, good and bad.

☐ I've prepared for tomorrow and all the unknowns it might bring.

Day 23

DON'T FORGET THE CHOCOLATE: MODERATION AND SELF-CONTROL

DON'T YOU JUST love having choices . . . chocolate or vanilla? Comedy or drama? Boxers or briefs?

But with so many choices, it's sometimes tough to exercise self-control. Our brains tend to default to the path of least resistance if we're overwhelmed with choices. There are so many possibilities that it's hard to gain self-control. Give in too many times and bad habits persist.

I've got a solution: Create boundaries for your behavior.

When you hear the word *boundaries*, you probably think of words like *rules*, *restrictions*, and *no fun*. But boundaries are anything but those things! Boundaries encourage self-love and freedom from self-destructive behavior.

A boundary in this sense is a healthy barrier between you and bad choices. It governs your behavior. It's a line you won't cross. It has a sign that reads STOP—NO GOING OVERBOARD HERE!

Suppose you're trying to kick a shopping habit. There are so many outlets bombarding you with products and "great values," from the mall and QVC to eBay and other online stores. You're constantly buying stuff, and most of it you don't really need. You're plunging into credit card debt as a result.

If you want to break your shopping habit and stop overspending, create the boundary that you can buy only one new item—such as a dress, shoes, or makeup— once a month. Stay within that constraint. Once you get used to doing that, your self-control gets stronger and your habit of overspending gets weaker.

Maybe you've gotten in the habit of having cocktails every night of the week and you want to cut back. You might set a boundary that you will have cocktails on Friday night only, and no more than two or three. Your desire will decrease over time. The more times you pass up the nightly cocktails, the easier it becomes to do so.

You can set boundaries at home and in relationships, too. Let's say you want time to go running but your family is always demanding your time. Be firm and tell them: six P.M. is Mom's (or Dad's) run time. So if you go for a run every day at six, your family will get used to it and won't try to hog your time with other demands.

Boundary setting applies at work, too. Maybe you want to stop being a workaholic. Make it a habit to leave work every day at five sharp. Eventually you'll learn to work smarter, not longer. Plus, your boss will learn not to dump late-night assignments on your desk at the last minute. You can empower yourself by setting boundaries.

One of the biggest areas where boundaries can help has to do with food and overeating. Know what I mean? If so, do what I do: Eat moderate portions and allow myself cheat meals.

LET ME ELABORATE. First, what do I mean by moderation? It's *not* stuffing yourself at all-you-can-eat buffets, taking jumbo servings at restaurants, or emptying a quart or more of chocolate ice cream. Moderation can involve an occasional splurge, but with portions kept under control.

If you can't quite picture what a moderate serving is, use the palm of your hand. Generally, no matter what the food (except salads—eat as much as you want of these), a normal serving fits nicely in the palm of your hand (not including your fingers!). Whether it's cereal, rice, pasta, or a slice of carrot cake, the palm of your hand is considered a medium (or moderate) portion.

So practice moderation; that's the first boundary.

Then plan your "cheat meals"—meals containing foods that are normally off-limits, such as cake, ice cream, and other fattening foods. When I say *cheat*, I'm talking about an individual meal or snack, not a whole day or week of cheating. A cheat meal is simply one where you add a *single* food to your plan that you might not otherwise eat, usually a carbohydrate. That cheat carb might be some pasta or a small roll. Or you might add a slice of pie to your meal.

You have to be careful with cheat meals, though. They can turn into cheat days, which turn into cheat weeks, and before long, your favorite all-you-can-eat-buffet restaurant will be sending you flowers and coupons. That's why I don't recommend cheat meals more than once a week at the most. Give me a couple of cheat meals a month and I'm completely happy. I believe in real-world dieting; I just want the option to eat what I want—occasionally.

Here's how I cheat. On Friday for a snack, I might treat myself to a cupcake, but only if I plan to have it. On a Sunday, if I go out for brunch with my girlfriends, I order scrambled eggs and veggies; then we all split an order of French toast for the cheat. (I spread mine with peanut butter to balance out my protein, carbs, and fat.) The entire brunch is a delicious scenario that gives me freedom, dietary leeway, and the enjoyment of a meal with friends. If I choose to indulge in an alcoholic beverage, I opt for clear liquor with soda water and lime. This eliminates all the extra sugars I could be consuming and doesn't leave me feeling bloated and crappy.

Set boundaries like these and you'll get control over food.

You have to realize that *you* are in control. Food, money, alcohol, drugs, other people, even negative emotions—none of these control you as long as you don't let them.

Simple boundary setting is one of the forces involved in building better habits and learning self-control. A little bit of self-control today could make you a big success tomorrow.

For Today

TODAY'S QUOTE

I have learned that I really do have discipline,
self-control, and patience. But they were given to me as a seed,
and it's up to me to choose to develop them.
—JOYCE MEYER

TODAY'S AFFIRMATION

_____

_____

_____

TODAY'S CHALLENGE

Write down one area in which lack of self-control is interfering with your ability to break bad habits: Finances? Gambling? Substance abuse? Weight and food? Inactivity? Some other habit or addiction?

Next, draw your line. Decide which behavior is not acceptable. Write down your boundaries so that they are easy to refer back to. Use the following fill-in-the-blank template to help you.

I will create a boundary around _____.

For example:
- Food
- Shopping
- Spending
- Drinking
- Overworking

Within those bounds, I will _____.

For example:
- Eat moderate portions.
- Allow myself cheat days.
- Buy only one new item a month.
- Deposit $100 a month in a savings account.
- Have only two cocktails a week.
- Put in an eight-hour workday, no more.
- Set aside a time just for me to meditate.
- Say no when I need to.

Having boundaries invites freedom, healthy living, and security into your life. They also teach *you* how to treat *you*.

Reflect. After you lived within your boundary for a couple of days, how did you feel? Satisfied? In control? Mentally and emotionally clearer?

Commit to setting boundaries and living within them. Experts say that self-control increases the more you practice it. Put another way: Self-control now becomes a positive new habit. You'll be in control of negative influences, not the other way around.

Today's Mental Goal:

_____

Today's Personal Goal:

_____

Today's Spiritual Goal:

_____

MY BADASS REFLECTIONS FOR TODAY

What are you most grateful for today?

Mentally: _____

Physically: _____

Spiritually: _____

What was the biggest success for you today?

Mentally: _____

Physically: _____

Spiritually: _____

What was the biggest challenge for you today? How did you overcome it?

Mentally: _____

Physically: _____

Spiritually: _____

What can you do tomorrow to make it a better day?

Mentally: _____

Physically: _____

Spiritually: _____

CHECKLIST

☐   I completed my habit change challenges.

☐   I made healthy choices today for my mind, body, and spirit.

☐   I've expressed my gratitude for today and all it brings, good and bad.

☐   I've prepared for tomorrow and all the unknowns it might bring.

Day 24
TURN SETBACKS INTO COMEBACKS

WITH THE MORNING sun beaming down on crystal-clear tropical waters, it was a perfect day to be riding the waves in Hawaii. Avid surfer Bethany Hamilton, then thirteen, was lying facedown on her board, dangling her left arm in the ocean and soaking up the sun. Suddenly something grabbed her arm and wouldn't let go, no matter how hard she tried to tug it away. Within seconds, the turquoise waters turned red with Bethany's blood. Powerless to escape, she felt her arm being ripped off just below the shoulder by a predator of the sea, a formidable fourteen-foot tiger shark.

Incredibly, just twenty-six days after the attack, Bethany was back in the water. Her goal hadn't changed. She wanted to be a professional surfer and didn't want to be frightened of the water. Without her left arm, Bethany faced many challenges.

No one knew if she could even balance on a board, let alone reach the levels of skill she'd achieved before. Now in her late twenties, she commands the waves and is one of the top-ranked professional female surfers in the world.

Bethany's story is an inspiring one of turning setbacks into comebacks.

You may not have had a limb chomped off by a shark, but you've no doubt experienced setbacks. Sometimes what throws us off track is our own fault: We drank too much at a party, we got laid off from a job, or we smoked the cigarette that triggered the relapse. At other times, the setback results from something out of control. For example, you accidentally injured your knee and thus can't work out for six weeks.

Setbacks can be as ordinary and annoying as a late-night work meeting that rules out an evening jog or as life-altering as a collapsed marriage or relationship, the loss of a job, a scary diagnosis, a bankruptcy, an injury, the death of a loved one, or a life-threatening disease. Lots of us have gone through purgatory or hell, but the question is: Did we make it back stronger than before?

Whether it was a large or a small setback, people going through and emerging from traumatic situations may feel stronger and more confident in themselves. They may develop a personal philosophy of life that uplifts them today and in the future. They may experience a change in priorities. For example, they want to enjoy the important things in life more—an illness might have this effect, for instance. Many people return to spiritual practices following traumatic experiences.

I see a lot of comebacks right under the roof of my gym. Geneen is a good example. She has had not one setback, but a series of setbacks, starting with a divorce five years ago that left her a single parent until her ex moved back to town. She then got involved in a string of destructive, abusive romantic relationships that eroded her self-trust and left her frightened. Over a year ago, she had major surgery. Compounding all of these situations was a demotion that lowered her income. She turned to food for comfort because she was so demoralized by her downward spiral.

Geneen kept asking herself: "Why me? Does someone have it in for me? Why is life so bad?"

I know all this because Geneen is a client of mine who got up enough nerve to start the hard work of changing her life by simply coming through the door of my gym. What brought her there was really her young son. She reached one of those turning points in which she knew she had to get her life together so she could provide a great life for him.

"I had easily gained seventy-five pounds," she said. "When it hit me that I was so overweight and sluggish that I couldn't do anything with my son, I decided to get help by joining CrossFit. I started exercising. At first it would take me twenty minutes to walk a mile. I was huffing and puffing. A month later, I started lifting weights. The weight came off, and the muscle came on. People who hadn't seen me didn't recognize me.

"Through my journey, I changed not just my body but also how I look at things. I look at the positives instead of the negatives, and life is great as a result. I got out of a rut I had dug for myself."

The ability to rebound from setbacks is called resilience. Resilient people realize that a setback is not the end of the road but merely a bend in the road. You crash only if you fail to make the turn.

Resilience comes from knowing yourself and how you respond to your environment. It affects how you handle setbacks and approach challenges. It keeps your thinking clear and focused during conflicts or stressful periods. Resilience helps you learn from past troubles and gain meaning from them. Responding effectively to bad stuff, from normal daily hassles to life-altering events, is at the heart of resilience.

So my question is: How can you become more resilient?

BECOME HEALTHIER. Resilient people consciously and actively take care of their health. So at the most basic level, you've got to have a healthy, strong body, developed through proper diet, regular exercise, and self-care. Good health gives you the energy, strength, mental power, and self-value to stand up to adversity, get past obstacles, and come out the other side better than you were before the setback.

During my own fitness transformation, it was obvious to me that if I wanted to go far in the field, I'd have to give up dearly beloved long-term habits such as drinking, smoking, and eating junk food full of fats and sugar. So I did.

Quiz: How Resilient Are You?

Here's another fun quiz to try in order to see how well you bounce back in life. Again, be honest!

1. If something difficult occurs in your life, which of these statements best reflects your response?

A. I will get through this, and I'll probably be stronger because of it in the end.

B. Why me?

C. I may never get over this.

2. When faced with a major challenge at work or in life, you tend to:

A. Do as much research as possible, devise a strategy, and follow through.

B. Gather information, but get overwhelmed, making it hard to take action.

C. Not spend much time thinking about it, and just go about your normal schedule.

3. When stressed out, your reaction is to:

A. Figure out what you can control in the situation and choose your response to the stressor.

B. Feel upset, try to choose your response, but generally just react.

C. Engage in unhealthy behaviors such as bingeing on food or alcohol.

4. Do you believe in something greater than yourself that can give you strength?

A. Yes.

B. Sometimes.

C. Never.

5. Are you in control of yourself with a healthy diet and regular exercise?

A. Yes, I lead a very healthy lifestyle.

B. A lot of the time, but it's hit or miss.

C. Not really; I just can't find the time.

6. How often do you laugh or find humor in situations?

A. I generally look on the bright side and laugh at life's little difficulties.

B. I try, but it can be hard.

C. I take tough things seriously; there's nothing funny about them.

7. How would you describe your ability to adapt to change?

A. I welcome change and see it as an important part of personal growth.

B. I try to accept change, but often find it uncomfortable.

C. I avoid change; it stresses me out too much.

8. When assigned a new task, you are:

A. Confident that I will succeed.

B. Not sure of the outcome, but I will try my best.

C. Worried that I will fail.

9. Do you have a support system in place—friends, family, or coworkers who can help you through a crisis?

A. Yes, I have close relationships with many people, and I can go to them for help at any time.

B. I have a few close confidants.

C. I'm somewhat of a loner and do not have many close friends.

10. If you experienced a profound emotional experience in the past, such as a death in the family, the loss of your job, or the end of a significant relationship, how long did it take you to bounce back?

A. A couple of months

B. A year or longer

C. I never got over it.

SCORING

For every A you circle, give yourself 5 points; for every B, 3 points; and every C, 1 point.

If you scored between 35 and 50 points, you are the king or queen of the bounce-back. You are able to put life's downs in perspective and move on in an emotionally healthy manner. You'd don't dwell on what went wrong, only on how to get it right the next time. You're the person who always sees the proverbial silver lining in every cloud. As for change, your motto is *Bring it on!*

If you scored between 20 and 34 points, your resiliency needs a little shoring up. The good thing is that you try hard at bouncing back, but sometimes you let a down mood slow you down. Try to remember that this, too, shall pass, and the sooner you get over something (with adequate time), the stronger your comeback will be.

If you scored between 10 and 19 points, you have a hard time returning to the comeback trail! Not to worry, though: You can strengthen your bounce-back muscles by reading inspiring stories of people who have overcome setbacks, surrounding yourself with a bigger circle of close friends, and learning to let go of hurts and disappointments. Keep reading. I've got more advice on how to bounce back successfully.

BUILD CONFIDENCE. Confidence is the belief that you'll be successful in a given situation, but it's not something we necessarily come by naturally, and it ebbs and flows. Few of us escape feelings of fear and self-doubt as we go about our lives.

You can choose your thoughts and therefore control your emotions. You have the natural ability to cancel any thought that makes you feel bad or depressed.

When negative mind chatter starts sounding off, replace it with a more empowering voice, such as "I can do this," "I'm strong today," "I'm grateful for what I have," or "I'm in control of my body and my life." Not only will you increase your confidence and success dramatically, but eventually those negative voices will get quieter and quieter as they recognize they have little influence on you.

As we go through this 30-day program, I realize you might not initially have the confidence that you can change your body and your life. That's okay! You don't have to believe it now to start it. Eventually, though, that belief will come when you see the results and feel the difference in your strength, energy, and overall well-being. You'll become a believer in your own power to be better than you've ever been. And others will notice!

MAKE LEMONADE. Remember the old saying "If life hands you lemons, make lemonade"? Or as Jimmy Buffett puts it: "If life gives you limes, make margaritas."

Both sayings describe resilience so well, and resilience is the reason so many people achieve great things despite what seem like insurmountable odds.

An example: You messed up a project at work. Instead of spending time wallowing in self-pity, ask yourself: What went well with the project? What can I do to avoid problems next time? Negative situations can turn into blessings—if you allow them to.

DON'T GET BITTER, GET BETTER. If you're like me and most other people, you can be your own worst critic. When you constantly beat yourself up, you get bitterer—and end up feeling bad about feeling bad.

Every thought you think becomes a command in your head, and your brain will carry out the commands it receives. So when you tell yourself things like "This is going to be hard," you're programming your brain to believe that whatever it is will be hard. That command gets embedded in your mind and will be carried out as programmed. Rather than thinking that something will be hard, say "I will enjoy this new challenge." See it, believe it, and then achieve it.

LOOK ON THE BRIGHT SIDE. Expect positive outcomes—not worst-case scenarios! Visualize the best-case scenario and let yourself feel connected to that outcome. This technique balances your thinking and creates positive expectations, which reinforces optimism and reduces anxiety.

TAKE ACTION. Take a certain degree of responsibility for the setback—no victim or whiner thinking. You might not be responsible for getting knocked down, but you are responsible for getting back up. Once you take responsibility for your part in the situation, you're ready to move forward and attain your next goal. Only those who act achieve their goals. Decide what you're going to do about the setback and focus on the solution.

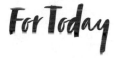

TODAY'S QUOTE

Persistence and resilience only come from having been given the chance to work through difficult problems.
—GEVER TULLEY

TODAY'S AFFIRMATION

_____

_____

_____

_____

TODAY'S CHALLENGE

Analyze one of the worst experiences you've ever had. What was it? Did you learn any valuable lessons? What were they? Write them in the space below.

_____

_____

Based on the insight you gained here, what can you do to build more resiliency?

_____

_____

Some suggestions to guide you:

☐ I will maintain a program of self-care. In any crisis, my mind and body need to be strong.

☐ I will not fall back on unhealthy behaviors like buying a carton of cigarettes, drinking a bottle of wine, or bingeing on doughnuts.

☐ I will seek the advice of my mentor to help prevent any future setbacks.

☐ I will maintain positivity and not let the setback put my life in reverse.

☐ I will seek the comfort of family and friends.

☐ I will remind myself that I haven't failed, I've just been thrown a curve ball.

☐ If needed, I will gain new knowledge and education that will help me take a new direction.

☐ I will give myself a certain timeline to heal prior to moving on.

☐ I will read comeback stories for inspiration.

Today's Mental Goal:

_____

Today's Personal Goal:

_____

Today's Spiritual Goal:

_____

MY RADASS REFLECTIONS FOR TODAY

What are you most grateful for today?

Mentally: _____

Physically: _____

Spiritually: _____

What was the biggest success for you today?

Mentally: _____

Physically: _____

Spiritually: _____

What was the biggest challenge for you today? How did you overcome it?

Mentally: _____

Physically: _____

Spiritually: _____

What can you do tomorrow to make it a better day?

Mentally: _____

Physically: _____

Spiritually: _____

CHECKLIST

☐   I completed my habit change challenges.

☐   I made healthy choices today for my mind, body, and spirit.

☐   I've expressed my gratitude for today and all it brings, good and bad.

☐   I've prepared for tomorrow and all the unknowns it might bring.

Day 25
TRAIN YOUR BRAIN

BESIDES YOUR BICEPS, triceps, abs, thighs, and other body parts, there's another other area of your body that needs a good workout: your brain. It is a use-it-or-lose-it organ. To really use it, you should engage in physical and mental workouts. The brain can influence the body and the mind through the power of thoughts, help you change bad habits, and inspire you to new heights of success.

How can you make all this happen?

YOUR BRAIN ON EXERCISE. Physical activity stimulates the growth of new brain cells and helps produce a crucial protein called *brain-derived neurotrophic factor*, or BDNF. This protein is responsible for forming new connections between brain cells and protects them from degeneration. So when you're building your muscles, you're also building your brain.

The benefits of exercise on the brain can be immediate, too. In a 2014 study at Stanford University, undergraduate students were asked to sit down and complete a short series of creativity tests that involved thinking up alternate uses for common household objects, such as a button or a spoon. Next, the students took the same tests while walking at a comfortable pace on a treadmill. For almost every student, creativity was boosted substantially when they walked. Most were able to generate 60 percent more new and practical uses for objects.

Why does physical exercise affect the brain so powerfully? The brain is a highly vascular organ, filled with blood vessels. Exercise gets blood pumping through those vessels, delivering oxygen and nutrients to brain cells for clearer thinking and optimum brain function.

Dancing—ballet, Zumba, ballroom, tap, line dancing; in fact, any form of dance that involves complex, coordinated movements—will power up your brain like nobody's business, too. As you concentrate and think through the moves, your brain starts making more dendrites (those bridges between brain cells that keep your brain young and active).

What matters, too, is that you exercise intensely. This finding was uncovered in research from the University of Kansas and published in the journal *PLOS ONE*. The investigators observed that any type of exercise improved brain function, but the intensity (level of effort) of the exercise appeared to matter more than the duration. In other words, to positively affect your brain, you need to push yourself a little harder than normal.

BUILD YOUR BRAINPOWER WITH POSITIVITY. You know all that positive, action-oriented thinking I've been talking about? Well, your brain loves it. Positivity prevents and alleviates stress and anxiety, both of which kill brain cells and prevent the creation of new ones.

And stress-relieving activities like relaxation and meditation? More good news. These techniques help improve memory. A 2007 study from the University of Pennsylvania suggests that meditation may train your brain to remember more. Twenty adults aged fifty-two to seventy with mild cognitive impairment (a precursor to Alzheimer's disease) practiced twelve minutes of meditation every day for eight weeks. Follow-up tests revealed increased blood flow to the region of the brain linked to learning and memory, and good brain circulation is known to boost memory.

FIND MORE LEARNING AND MENTAL CHALLENGES. The brain loves to learn, and it loves a challenge. Both stimulate the growth of new brain cells. The harder the challenge, the stronger the brain gets and the longer new brain cells survive. The point of having a brain is precisely to learn and to adapt to challenging, new environments. This does not mean doing crossword puzzles every day. Your brain gets stronger when you challenge it with novel activities. Some examples:

* Studying a new language
* Learning to play a musical instrument
* Returning to school
* Taking up any new hobby that has a steep learning curve and requires mental focus, such as sailing, painting, or woodworking

TRAVEL AND EXPLORE. Ruts and routines can dull your brain. Try to do something completely different and fun each week to shake your brain out of its complacency. Some examples: Go to places you've never visited, take a new route home from the movies, explore an unfamiliar shop, or join a book club. Afterward, challenge your memory by trying to recall as many details of your experience as possible.

DEVELOP AND MAINTAIN STIMULATING FRIENDSHIPS. We are social animals, and we need social interaction. Socializing forces your brain to use much of its frontal lobe region, which is responsible for problem solving. Whether you're meeting new people at the gym or chatting with old friends over lunch, social activities flex your mental muscle. So to stay sharp, stay social.

LAUGH OFTEN AND MUCH. Laughter boosts your memory. The reason has to do with the stress hormone cortisol. Levels spike when you're tense and stressed out.

Chronically high levels of cortisol can harm your heart, liver, stomach, and brain. Excess cortisol specifically can damage neurons in the hippocampus, the region of the brain responsible for forming new memories. So look for more ways to laugh. Read funny books, watch comedies, and check out cartoons.

PLAY BRAIN GAMES. I've got the coolest solution to building your mental toughness and having fun at the same time. Play board games! In 2013, a group of French researchers published a fascinating study of people who were avid board-game players, in order to see if the games had any positive effects on brain skills. Here's what happened. About twenty years ago, the researchers selected 3,675 participants with no memory, thinking, or dementia-type problems. Among them, about 32 percent were regular board-game players. The researchers followed up with these folks twenty years later. Lo and behold, the risk of dementia was 15 percent lower in board-game players than in nonplayers.

What does this mean to you and me? Pull out your Scrabble boards, your Trivial Pursuit game, or your Stratego and start playing. All of these games and others are excellent for keeping your brain alert and your memory sharp.

Sudoku, chess, bridge, and crossword puzzles are also helpful. They build verbal skills and keep your brain stimulated and powered up. Chess in particular improves your power of concentration, perception, and reasoning. Phone apps and computer games can improve cognitive performance and short-term working memory, too. But be careful not to overuse technology, because if we constantly get distracted by it, our mental performance can worsen.

The secrets to lifelong mental toughness involve some pretty simple changes in lifestyle and outlook. Even if you apply only a handful of my suggestions, you'll be well on your way to building a superfit mind.

For Today

Our minds influence the key activity of the brain, which then influences everything; perception, cognition, thoughts and feelings, personal relationships; they're all a projection of you.
—DEEPAK CHOPRA

TODAY'S AFFIRMATION

_____

_____

_____

TODAY'S CHALLENGE

Shake things up today with one or all of these activities:

Read a magazine that you would never read normally pick up. Your brain needs to see and experience new things to stimulate fresh perspectives.

Rewire your brain for happiness. Today write down and describe in detail the most meaningful experiences you've had in the past forty-eight hours. Do this every day. Research shows that this simple habit rewires your brain and improves its ability to create feelings of happiness.

Practice meditation. Meditation is good for the brain. Anyone can meditate, and it takes only five to ten minutes a day. Here's how:

- Find a quiet spot without distractions or disruptions. Either lie down on a mat or sit in a comfortable chair. Close your eyes.
- Relax your body by systematically tensing muscle groups while inhaling and then breathing away tension on the exhale.
- Once your body is relaxed, bring your attention to your breathing, particularly noticing your exhale. As you breathe out, let go of thoughts—whatever is in your mind. If you get lost in a thought—from planning your next shopping trip or revisiting a memory to going over a problem at work—just let it go on the next exhalation.
- Or you might choose to focus on a relaxing image such as a mountaintop or a sandy beach. Whenever other thoughts intrude in your mind, focus on that image.
- After five or ten minutes have passed, open your eyes and notice how you feel.

Today's Mental Goal:

_____

Today's Personal Goal:

_____

Today's Spiritual Goal:

_____

MY BADASS REFLECTIONS FOR TODAY

What are you most grateful for today?

Mentally: _____

Physically: _____

Spiritually: _____

What was the biggest success for you today?

Mentally: _____

Physically: _____

Spiritually: _____

What was the biggest challenge for you today? How did you overcome it?

Mentally: _____

Physically: _____

Spiritually: _____

What can you do tomorrow to make it a better day?

Mentally: _____

Physically: _____

Spiritually: _____

CHECKLIST

☐   I completed my habit change challenges.

☐   I made healthy choices today for my mind, body, and spirit.

☐   I've expressed my gratitude for today and all it brings, good and bad.

☐   I've prepared for tomorrow and all the unknowns it might bring.

Day 26
HAVE SUCCESSFUL
FAILURES

TODAY LET'S TALK about the F-word. I mean *failure*. (What did you think I meant?)

Just because I've accomplished so much doesn't mean it came without failure or trials. I first met and fell in love with failure in my twenties, when I wanted to kick drugs and smoking. It was tough. I failed a lot. But every time I failed, I gained insight into what wasn't working. Failing taught me that I had to reduce my exposure to smoking triggers like drinks after work and my drug-taking triggers like certain people and situations.

I met failure again at the 2015 USA Weightlifting American Open, where I lost big-time. But guess what? Failure helped me refocus and launch two important projects: this book and my Christmas Abbott app.

Failure is okay.

If you don't think so, check out some of the most famous failures in history:

J. K. Rowling, who penned the Harry Potter series, says that an early failed marriage and hitting financial rock bottom as a single mother gave her the freedom and motivation to write.

Michael Jordan was once cut from his high school basketball team.

Babe Ruth, in pursuing the home run record, also landed the record for most strikeouts, totaling 1,330.

Winston Churchill lost every election for public office until he became prime minister of Great Britain.

Unlike these famous failures, many of us avoid the prospect of failure. We're so focused on *not* failing that we forget about success, or we let failure sideline us with depression over what we see as missteps or mistakes. Or we plain give up if we don't nail something perfectly the first time.

Failure is only true failure if you quit. I know what you're thinking: *I didn't hit my goal, so I failed*. But that isn't true. If you attempt something only one time, it's likely you won't succeed. Success is built on the knowledge created from failures. We need failed attempts to show us the way to success! If you go forward and try something, without quite hitting your mark or goal, I consider that a *successful failure*.

Here's how I look at failure:

LEARN FROM FAILURE. Failure is a temporary and necessary step on the way to where you want to be. Think about toddlers learning to walk. When they fall down, would you say, "You really messed up"? Or would you say, "Good for you, you walked a couple of steps"? Yet when we fall down (blow the sales opportunity, get fired from a job, screw up a relationship, and so forth), we tell ourselves, "I failed!" Okay, but when you do "fail," recover quickly by asking, "What can I learn from this? What worked and what didn't? How can I do it better next time?" Then follow the toddler's example—get up and try again.

Unless you learn from failure, you're bound to repeat your mistakes. But if you learn some key fundamentals from your failure, this gets you close to success in life. Henry Ford put it best: "Failure is simply the opportunity to begin again, this time more intelligently."

GROW FROM FAILURE. If you do get back up again and again and learn from the failure, you'll grow and improve. Maybe that toddler turns out to be a world-class runner. Or that job you got fired from paves the way to a better opportunity at which you can excel. That failed relationship taught you what you really wanted from a partner. You experience success through failure. It allows us to know what we really want and how badly we really want it. Without failure, we don't understand what our current abilities truly are and how to harvest our inner beast to get what we desire. If you never fail, you've missed a lot of opportunities—especially the kinds of opportunities most often disguised as challenges.

GET OVER THE FEAR OF FAILURE. A lot of us are too hung up on results. We're afraid of failing, so we stay stuck and overwhelmed. Or we think we have to be perfect. Life is not a game of perfection. Trying to be perfect can keep you from trying new and untested methods for reaching your goals. Striving for perfection is fine, but expecting it is unrealistic. It's better to strive for progress and bold, resolute action in the direction of your goals.

These feelings are common when you set out to do something big or even just exciting. Fear is a naturally protective mechanism when your physical survival is an issue. But you're not going to die if you blow a sales call, get dumped, or are passed over for a promotion. Fear of failure will hold you back from pursuing your dreams, accomplishing your goals, or making the impossible possible. Snap out of this overwhelmed feeling by not worrying about the outcome. It's better to focus on things you can control, such as the effort you put in; then great results will flow.

So today I wish you failure—lots of it, faster, and often. If you learn from it, grow from it, and don't fear it, you'll achieve exhilarating success.

Now go F-word yourself toward your dreams!

···

For Today

TODAY'S QUOTE

I have not failed. I've just found 10,000 ways that won't work.
—THOMAS A. EDISON

TODAY'S AFFIRMATION

_____

_____

_____

TODAY'S CHALLENGES

Try one or both of these activities today:

Sit down in a quiet place. Reflect on a few times you failed. Then list everything positive you learned from your failures. Now turn those lessons into action steps toward your goals.

Feeling down about a failure but having trouble learning from it? Get up from your computer or work space right now and take a walk. The longer, the better (try the walking meditation on page 34). Walking was a favorite technique used by Albert Einstein to help solve problems he was working on.

Today's Mental Goal:

_____

Today's Personal Goal:

_____

Today's Spiritual Goal:

_____

MY BADASS REFLECTIONS FOR TODAY

What are you most grateful for today?

Mentally: _____

Physically: _____

Spiritually: _____

What was the biggest success for you today?

Mentally: _____

Physically: _____

Spiritually: _____

What was the biggest challenge for you today? How did you overcome it?

Mentally: _____

Physically: _____

Spiritually: _____

What can you do tomorrow to make it a better day?

Mentally: _____

Physically: _____

Spiritually: _____

CHECKLIST

☐   I completed my habit change challenges.

☐   I made healthy choices today for my mind, body, and spirit.

☐   I've expressed my gratitude for today and all it brings, good and bad.

☐   I've prepared for tomorrow and all the unknowns it might bring.

Day 27
DEVELOP HEALTHY OBSESSIONS

I HAVE AN addictive personality. Fortunately I was able to channel my bad addictions into positive ones—namely CrossFit, competitions, and fitness in general. I sort of jumped head over heels into all this and never looked back.

I discovered that having a goal to stop doing something unhealthy is not nearly as effective as making a goal that involves doing something new. If you have a bad habit to overcome, focus on creating a new behavior in that situation—which is what I did. When you replace a bad habit with a good one, it's almost like starting your life all over again. You start telling yourself, "Whew, I don't have to worry about *that* anymore."

Training and competition ultimately became a way of life for me—just good, positive energy and healthy obsessions. It's not possible to overdose on them.

Quiz: Do You Have an Addictive Personality?

Take this quiz to find out. Acknowledging life issues is the first step toward resolving them in a positive way.

1. Do you enjoy activities such as gambling or purchasing lottery tickets?

A. Yes, love the rush.
B. It's fun.
C. Every so often.
D. Nah.

2. You feel stuffed after the main course. Will you go for the delicious dessert afterward?

A. Absolutely.
B. Thinking about it.
C. Not sure.
D. No way.

3. How often are you on social media?

A. I'm constantly checking it and/or posting stuff on Facebook and Instagram.
B. I'm on it only if I'm bored.
C. Not too often.
D. I seldom look at it.

4. When you try something for the first time and find you really like it, how do you feel afterward?

A. Obsessed—I can't wait to do it again.
B. Enjoyment—but then it leaves my mind for a while.
C. It was a good experience. I may or may not do it again.
D. No feelings, really.

5. Do you routinely crave a physical substance, such as cigarettes, alcohol, drugs, or food?

A. A lot!
B. Often.
C. Occasionally.
D. Rarely or never.

6. At least one of your parents displayed some sort of addictive behavior (alcohol or drug abuse, smoking, compulsive gambling, and so forth).

A. No doubt about it.
B. Perhaps.
C. Not sure.
D. No way.

7. You have some bad habits that you hide from your friends and family.

A. Yes, all the time.

B. Sometimes.

C. Rarely.

D. Never.

8. Your love of excitement and risk taking (driving fast, having sexual flings, doing drugs, and so on) is:

A. Off the charts—I am a thrill seeker and an adrenaline junkie.

B. Moderate.

C. I've taken risks, but not very often.

D. Nonexistent; I avoid risk taking and risky behavior.

9. You are more likely to make snap decisions without considering the long-term consequences.

A. Yep, that's me.

B. Every now and then.

C. Seldom.

D. Nah.

10. You tend to lack self-control.

A. Yep, that's me.

B. Every now and then.

C. Seldom.

D. Nah.

SCORING

If your answers were mostly A's (5 or more), you have a highly addictive personality type. You may even have more than one close relative that has a similar personality. You have a very hard time grasping, accepting, or appreciating the concept of moderation. The good thing is that by taking this quiz, you've acknowledged a potential problem—which means you're already on track to change it.

If your answers were mostly B's and C's, you enjoy a few potentially addictive things or activities, but you exercise enough self-control to not let them get out of hand.

If your answers were mostly D's, you're squeaky clean in your lack of excess. You're not impulsive in the least and live your life without artificial "boosts" in the form of brain chemicals, mood stimulants, or other bad habits.

I will do them forever. I love to train. I love to push my body and mind. To me, the weights are representative of some of the struggles we go through in life. You push against those struggles and try to be victorious over them.

I wouldn't give it up or trade it for the world. Without working out, I don't think

I'd be as energetic or as confident as I am now. It basically just makes me feel good, even if I'm not having the greatest day.

Researchers have known about the addictive qualities of exercise for decades. Exercisers and athletes get hooked on endorphins, the body's natural painkillers that surge into the brain and bloodstream during exercise. This is the runner's high you hear about—a feeling of well-being that comes with physical activity.

How about you? What healthy obsessions do you have, or what activities could become your healthy obsessions?

Yours do not have to be exercise. They could be a hobby you love but haven't spent time developing. Examples include painting, refinishing furniture, singing, playing a musical instrument, needlework, a sport, arts and crafts, dancing . . . the list is endless.

And guess what? You could turn your hobby into a life's work. A great example is housewife Kim Lavine. In 2001 she started making "spa therapy" pillows as gifts for her children's teachers. The pillows can be warmed in the microwave and tucked in bed with you to give a nice neck massage. She used a corn kernel filling and assembled them on her kitchen table in Grand Haven, Michigan. About the same time, her husband lost his job, prompting Kim to turn her hobby into income.

She patented the idea and began peddling the pillows from her truck. They were so popular that she started selling them at mall kiosks. Within just two years, Kim's Wuvit pillow was sold in national chains, including Saks Fifth Avenue, Macy's, and Bed Bath & Beyond, and by 2006, the product had generated more than $1 million in sales.

Kim then branched out, producing pajamas and a whole line of home lifestyle products. She shared her success secrets in a book called *Mommy Millionaire: How I Turned My Kitchen Table Idea into a Million Dollars and How You Can, Too!* You never know where a healthy obsession may lead.

When you have a healthy obsession, you will:

- Experience more good moods.
- Have a more positive outlook on life.

- Overcome some bad habits and replace them with healthy ones.
- Love yourself more.
- Feel more energized.
- Be proud of yourself.
- Feel confident in your abilities.
- Discover a way to turn your hobby into a business or second career.
- Feel within reach of your dreams and goals.

But if you're still working on developing your own healthy obsession, that's okay. You'll find it. Just keep trying. A simple thing like walking could be your turning point. If you care enough about yourself to take a walk every day, it could completely change your perspective—even your life.

Along the way, be sure to balance your healthy obsession with your personal life, or else your obsession becomes unhealthy. One simple way I balance my workouts with my personal life is to get them done first thing in the morning, so that it's the first thing off my plate.

Enjoy your healthy obsession, but don't lose sight of why you're doing it. Do it for yourself and you'll never be disappointed with what you achieve.

I think, too, that having one healthy obsession—say, exercising or pursuing a great hobby—helps you take control of other areas of your life. Just think: If you can accomplish just one healthy obsession, what else can you change? Get out of debt? Lose those last few pounds? Become more organized? One healthy obsession empowers you to develop other healthy obsessions.

We all deserve a successful life, and you will succeed as long as you believe you can do it. So always work on replacing bad habits with healthy new ones that elevate your life. It's impossible to be down on yourself when you're doing things you love.

...

For Today

Today is life—the only life you are sure of. Make the most of today. Get interested in something. Shake yourself awake. Develop a hobby. Let the winds of enthusiasm sweep through you. Live today with gusto.
—DALE CARNEGIE

TODAY'S AFFIRMATION

_____

_____

TODAY'S CHALLENGE

Find your healthy obsession. Based on my experience, I have some tips for finding and pursuing a healthy obsession. Choose an activity that:

- You can do it for at least thirty minutes daily.
- You can enjoy alone, or at least don't have to rely on others to pursue it.
- You feel it has physical, mental, or spiritual value.
- You're confident you can improve your performance in if you keep at it.
- You can do it without criticizing yourself.
- You feel great, amazing, and empowered after finishing it.
- You are impassioned when pursuing it.

Next, list activities that fit most of these criteria. Now go out and do them!

_____

_____

Today's Mental Goal:

_____

Today's Personal Goal:

_____

Today's Spiritual Goal:

_____

MY BADASS REFLECTIONS FOR TODAY

What are you most grateful for today?

Mentally: _____

Physically: _____

Spiritually: _____

What was the biggest success for you today?

Mentally: _____

Physically: _____

Spiritually: _____

What was the biggest challenge for you today? How did you overcome it?

Mentally: _____

Physically: _____

Spiritually: _____

What can you do tomorrow to make it a better day?

Mentally: _____

Physically: _____

Spiritually _____:

CHECKLIST

☐   I completed my habit change challenges.

☐   I made healthy choices today for my mind, body, and spirit.

☐   I've expressed my gratitude for today and all it brings, good and bad.

☐   I've prepared for tomorrow and all the unknowns it might bring.

Day 28

TAKE CONTROL OF ROLLER-COASTER EMOTIONS

I'VE DEFINITELY HAD periods of time where sad emotions overtook me. Activities I loved went out the window. My fit lifestyle disappeared. I gave my power away to depression and anxiety.

I just didn't give a shit.

But when it really hit me that my emotions were denying me my own success and happiness, I snapped out of the funk and pressed PLAY.

Often we allow negative emotions to shape our thoughts and priorities. But to be successful in every aspect of life, we've got to take control of the negativity, make conscious, healthy choices, and guide the course of our lives—in our careers, finances, health, and relationships—in the direction of our dreams. This is easier said than done, though. So how can we take control of roller-coaster emotions to continue reshaping our lives?

Be grateful. When you begin to be grateful for what's right in your life rather than looking at what's wrong—you own your own home, you're basically healthy, you have people who love you, and so on—you will immediately move into a great mood. Seriously! Make a list of everything you're grateful for, and add to it weekly. Post your list where you can see it every day. Notice how your mood stabilizes and changes for the better.

Act, don't react. Shit happens, and it happens to all of us. It's how you respond to the shit that that counts. You see, we tend to go around assuming that things are done to us. "My boyfriend makes me mad," "My boss makes me nervous," "My mother drives me crazy." Sure, those people may be the triggers, but it is our thoughts, directed and controlled by us, that create the anger, anxiety, guilt, depression, and other unpleasant emotions. The point is that we often make or break our experiences.

The best antidote here is to step back and put things into perspective. We never really know what's going on in someone else's life, do we? That person could have just received a crushing medical diagnosis, lost a loved one, or been fired from a job. I heard something on the news that speaks to this. A young husband was rushing in traffic to get to the hospital to see his newborn. He cut another guy off in traffic. That guy exploded in road rage and shot and killed the young father. Had the driver known the father's situation, perhaps this tragedy would never have happened.

You get to make a choice about how an incident or a person is going to affect you. You can rerun the encounter over in your head or you can decide to let it go. Odds are the rude waiter or crazy driver is not stewing about you. He or she has already moved on.

Once you realize that other people's actions and reactions are out of your control, you can free yourself from this bondage. While letting go is easier said than done, I've found myself bouncing back more quickly than in the past after taking this advice to heart. So stop assuming that things are being done to you or that you're a victim. FIFO whether you're overreacting to situations, and respond rationally. Just the way you think about and approach a situation can make all the difference.

Use negative emotions for positive change. In many ways, unpleasant emotions are like the security system in your home. They warn you that something's wrong with your life. If you're frustrated over your unfulfilling job, that's a sign that you need to look for a new one. If you're depressed over the fifty extra pounds you're carrying on your body, that's a sign that you need to change your lifestyle. If you're anxious and stressed in your relationship, this may be a sign that you need to dump your boyfriend or girlfriend. We can use negative emotions such as anger, frustration, jealousy, or anxiety as motivation to improve our lives and turn them into achievement.

Stay aware of how you're feeling. Emotions are energy, and they influence how you come across. If you're angry, depressed, or lonely, your body language will relay a lack of confidence and joy, your tone of voice will lack confidence, and your conversation will have little self-assurance—all of which will block your path to success. If your demeanor keeps going south when you need to be at your best, find a way to boost yourself back up (try exercise—the greatest antidepressant ever invented). Because if you don't, all you'll do is perpetuate the problem.

We can choose to wallow in misery or go about a positive life. If you aren't happy with your life, then you and your thoughts have the power to change it! Positive emotions and actions will follow. Once you're aware of how this works, you can start to use it deliberately to get what you want from life.

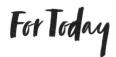

TODAY'S QUOTE

Every day we have plenty of opportunities to get angry, stressed or offended. But what you're doing when you indulge these negative emotions is giving something outside yourself power over your happiness. You can choose to not let little things upset you.

—JOEL OSTEEN

TODAY'S AFFIRMATION

_____

_____

_____

TODAY'S CHALLENGE

When we think irrationally, we provoke negative emotions—which in turn may produce a chain reaction of destructive behavior. Example:

"I screwed up that project royally; I'm so stupid." (This is a thought.)
"I am so bummed and depressed." (The thought leads to negative emotions.)
"I'm going out to get drunk." (The negative emotions lead to negative behaviors.)

See how these strings of thoughts, emotions, and behavior link to each other?

Your thoughts create your feelings, and feelings produce actions or inaction.

In your journal, write each of the self-defeating thoughts, feelings, and actions that you've experienced today. Another example:

1. "I blew an important sales call; I'm so incompetent."

2. I'm disappointed and depressed, so . . .

3. I ate an entire pizza at lunch.

Using the chart below, let's discover what sorts of negative thoughts are creating your bad feelings—and what to do about them.

COLUMN A:	COLUMN B:	COLUMN C:
Write down the negative thoughts, emotions, and actions: "I blew an important sales call; I'm so incompetent. I'm disappointed and depressed so I ate an entire pizza at lunch."	Identify and label any irrational thoughts for what they are. For example: You've had lots of successful sales calls. You can't be incompetent. In other words, give the thoughts a reality check. See if they are true, rather than just assuming "It must be true because I feel it."	Counter these negative thoughts with positive, rational responses. Examples: *I may have failed at one sales call (or maybe a few), but that doesn't make me a failure, nor does it make me incompetent.*

Today's Mental Goal:

_____

Today's Personal Goal:

_____

Today's Spiritual Goal:

_____

MY BADASS REFLECTIONS FOR TODAY

What are you most grateful for today?

   Mentally: _____

   Physically: _____

   Spiritually: _____

What was the biggest success for you today?

   Mentally: _____

   Physically: _____

   Spiritually: _____

What was the biggest challenge for you today? How did you overcome it?

   Mentally: _____

   Physically: _____:

Spiritually: _____

What can you do tomorrow to make it a better day?

Mentally: _____

Physically: _____

Spiritually: _____

CHECKLIST

☐   I completed my habit change challenges.

☐   I made healthy choices today for my mind, body, and spirit.

☐   I've expressed my gratitude for today and all it brings, good and bad.

☐   I've prepared for tomorrow and all the unknowns it might bring.

Day 29
SOLIDIFY INTENTION

ON A REGULAR basis, I make a list of my personal intentions, using positive, affirmative words. Some examples: *I will do my best and train hard for my upcoming competition. I will serve my clients with joy. I will grow my business. I will honor my family.*

The reason I do this is simple: Making an intention is like taking aim at the targets or goals I've set for myself. It gives a focused direction to everything I do, and I find myself automatically making choices that expedite my reaching my goals.

But just because you solidify your intentions like this doesn't mean your goals will be achieved. If you've got some reservations or negative thoughts lurking under the surface of your mind, they can make the arrow of your intention miss the mark. This is true whether your intention is to attract money, love, health, and other positives into your life.

These counterproductive feelings are what psychologists call *limiting beliefs*—thoughts we have in our heads that subtly hold us back from our dreams. One of the limiting beliefs I adopted at an early age was that I wouldn't amount to anything or do anything important or even impressive. No one around me had any high hopes for me, so I had no high hopes for myself. That belief had a way of manifesting itself. As a result, I was always making a mess of anything I tried.

EXAMINE YOURSELF. Socrates famously said, "An unexamined life is not worth living." It is only through a close examination of ourselves that we can identify what we truly want and want to become. Okay, what are your limiting beliefs? What is holding you back from reaching your maximum potential?

Maybe you believe that you can't achieve the body you've always dreamed of. You've got to reprogram your belief to think of yourself as fit and attractive, seeing it in your mind, and you'll be well on your way toward achieving that goal. Or maybe you believe you can't make more money than you're making now. You've got to start thinking that you can become wealthy. Own the belief that you can, and you'll reach your financial goals. Consciously shift away from limiting beliefs, and you can move toward more control over your life.

STOP USING THE WORDS *DON'T* OR *CAN'T*. The brain creates images of the words that follow these words. Replace every *don't* with *do* and every *can't* with *can* and see the difference in your results. Say to yourself, "I can start my own business . . . create my own blog . . . go into politics," instead of "I can't do any of those things." Your thoughts have a structure that you can alter. You can transform how you think. Doing so provides life-changing possibilities because your mind is so powerful.

OVERRIDE BAD STUFF. Once you've identified and reprogrammed the beliefs you feel may be holding you back, the next step is to override these feelings with explicit definitions of the behavior you intend to perform and what attitude or mindset will accompany that behavior. For example, you might tell yourself that you will work a full eight hours to complete an important project today. You don't say, "I will try"—there's no *trying* because that word implies doubt; you set your intention by saying, "I will"—period! (Affirmations are an effective way to set and solidify intention, too, and I cover those on day 2.) Setting your intention then becomes like an automatic missile guidance system in your head that exerts self-direction and purposeful action.

Attach positive emotion, enthusiasm, and desire to your intention. When you want something so strongly and you align with it, the universe works with you to bring it in.

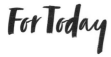

TODAY'S QUOTE

We either live with intention or exist by default.
—KRISTIN ARMSTRONG

TODAY'S AFFIRMATION

_____

_____

_____

_____

_____

Set an intention to do something that means the world to you.

Write down your intentions, beginning with the words *I intend to . . .*

As with affirmations, post your intentions where you can see them. When you live your intentions, you'll find those you're automatically kinder to yourself, you'll make choices aligned with those intentions, and you'll naturally make progress toward your goals.

Next spend at least five minutes every day reciting your intentions to yourself. You can do this exercise anytime, anywhere, but it's especially helpful at times when you feel stressed or believe that you might stray from your goals.

Today's Mental Goal:

_____

Today's Personal Goal:

_____

Today's Spiritual Goal:

_____

MY BADASS REFLECTIONS FOR TODAY

What are you most grateful for today?

Mentally: _____

Physically: _____

Spiritually: _____

What was the biggest success for you today?

Mentally: _____

Physically: _____

Spiritually: _____

What was the biggest challenge for you today? How did you overcome it?

Mentally: _____

Physically: _____

Spiritually: _____

What can you do tomorrow to make it a better day?

Mentally: _____ :

Physically: _____ :

Spiritually: _____

CHECKLIST

☐   I completed my habit change challenges.

☐   I made healthy choices today for my mind, body, and spirit.

☐   I've expressed my gratitude for today and all it brings, good and bad.

☐   I've prepared for tomorrow and all the unknowns it might bring.

Day 30

CLIMB THE UNCLIMBABLE

THERE IS A steep vertical cliff in Yosemite National Park called El Capitan that extends straight up, about 3,000 feet from base to summit; it is considered the largest granite rock face in the world. With dangerous cracks and narrow ledges, El Capitan was once thought to be unclimbable, but a mountaineer named Warren Harding was dead set on doing it. He put together a team and chose a route called the Nose on the prow of the massive cliff. On November 12, 1958, Harding and two others, George Whitmore and Wayne Merry, scrambled victoriously onto the summit. They had climbed the unclimbable, and today El Capitan is one of the world's favorite challenges for rock climbers.

The moral of this story is that there is no goal that cannot be met, no habit that cannot be broken, no dream that cannot come true. With faith in yourself (and some hard-core grit!), you can climb your way to success.

The climb happens little by little, and you don't have to reach the pinnacle of success before you begin enjoying it. Every time you eat a healthy vegetable, take a walk around the block, or halt a bad habit even for a day, you earn yourself a little more internal credibility. After a few weeks—or even after the 30 days we've been together—the alternatives like pigging out on the couch or getting drunk at night or giving up on stuff you tried to start don't seem worth it anymore. With every step, you gain success.

I get many letters from people who share their success stories with me. Many people want to give up, even on life. Once I did a video with *Self* magazine in which I told my own story. The gist of my testimonial was "One day I decided I was worth living for."

So many people reached out to me after seeing that video—and decided they were worth it, too. Some went to counselors; others joined self-help groups; many resumed their gym memberships. These stories moved me so much that I just crumpled in a chair and cried tears of gratitude and thankfulness.

I don't know where you are in your own journey, but I maintain that you are worth it, and you can do anything you make up your mind you want to do. You can achieve a healthy, fit body. You can climb high in your job. You can build a successful business of your own. You can be happy. The more you climb and the higher you climb, the more power you have to succeed at whatever you want to change and to conquer any self-control challenge you face.

How do you keep that momentum going? How do you climb the unclimbable?

PUT IN THE WORK. People have often said to me: "You're so lucky." I'm not lucky. I worked hard to get what I've earned. Sure, I've moaned in the mornings that I didn't want to get up and train, but all that resulted was I felt grumpy, and I still didn't get any training done. The progress we all seek comes from putting in the work each day. Just because you don't feel that great doesn't mean you can't accomplish anything. We all have days where we cannot be bothered to do anything—we feel tired, bored, or unmotivated. But choosing to put the work in anyway—even if it's just twenty or thirty minutes—will mean you'll move faster along your path and get more done.

This "philosophy" of putting in the work each day, regardless of how you feel, can be applied to all facets of your life—your training, your nutrition, your job, even your relationships. Imagine how much stress and guilt we could remove from our lives if we just worked hard every single day! If you keep at it, you'll see improvements in your body, mind, and mood, while reinforcing some positive new habits. And you'll be motivated to set new goals to keep your momentum going.

PUT YOURSELF FIRST. No matter how crazy things get with demands from work, family, school, and so forth, make yourself a priority. I know this is hard for women especially, because we're always concerned about taking care of others first. This isn't a bad thing, but it can be problematic when you don't value your well-being enough to put it at the top of your priority list. How can you take care of others properly unless you take care of yourself first? Start looking at your diet and workouts as rewards. A healthy lifestyle is a lot more fun when you approach it from a healthy, positive state of mind.

PREPARE METICULOUSLY TO INCREASE YOUR CHANCES OF SUCCESS. Make grocery lists, write out your daily schedule and goals, and prep your mind through positive self-talk, visualization, and attitude adjustments. Preparation is a habit— and probably a cornerstone for everything in life. The brave mountaineers I mentioned earlier spent forty-seven days over sixteen months setting up their route with bolts, ropes, hardware, food, and camping gear to prepare for their climb. Preparation is the catalyst for self-discipline. It builds self-confidence, and it's tough to succeed without it.

FIND SOMETHING PEOPLE THINK IS IMPOSSIBLE AND THEN DO IT. I don't know what that is for you. A run for public office? Starting a business? Climbing a mountain? Anything is possible, but the hint of impossibility creeps into our heads from outside forces. People, messages, images, sounds, and media overwhelm us nearly every minute of our lives. We become that to which we are exposed, unfortunately. I was a druggie because I hung out with druggies. To combat this negative overload, spend time by yourself, away from those messages and people who bring you down and essentially reclaim new visions of what you *can* do.

You are a success the moment you start your climb to success. You don't have to wait until you have the money to join a gym or until your life stresses are less or until New Year's. You can be a success right now . . . so start living life to the fullest.

For Today

TODAY'S QUOTE

You don't climb mountains without a team, you don't climb mountains without being fit, you don't climb mountains without being prepared, and you don't climb mountains without balancing the risks and rewards. And you never climb a mountain by accident—it has to be intentional.
—MARK UDALL

TODAY'S AFFIRMATION

_____

_____

_____

_____

_____

What are your mountains? Are there things you'd like to do or achieve in
life—big, bold, crazy things? Or are there some tough struggles you need to
overcome? These are your mountains; we need them because they make us
stronger. List your mountains here.

_____

_____

_____

Start the climb. How will you prepare for the climb? As you face your
mountains, maybe you need some mentors, friends, or family members to
help you or provide the encouragement you need to make the climb.

    List your climb strategies below, perhaps using some of the techniques and
ideas you've gain over these past 30 days:

_____

_____

_____

Keep climbing to the mountaintop. During one of your daily meditations, see
yourself pushing forward, living that impossible dream, or overcoming a really
tough journey. Keep going. You may not be able to see above the tree line yet,
but just keep climbing. It will come. And the view you see will be incredible.
When you come to the top of your mountain one day, you'll be thankful for
the climb you had to take.

Today's Mental Goal:

_____

Today's Personal Goal:

_____

Today's Spiritual Goal:

_____

MY BADASS REFLECTIONS FOR TODAY

What are you most grateful for today?

Mentally: _____

Physically: _____

Spiritually: _____

What was the biggest success for you today?

Mentally: _____

Physically: _____

Spiritually: _____

What was the biggest challenge for you today? How did you overcome it?

Mentally: _____

Physically: _____

Spiritually: _____

What can you do tomorrow to make it a better day?

Mentally: _____

Physically: _____

Spiritually: _____

CHECKLIST

☐ I completed my habit change challenges.

☐ I made healthy choices today for my mind, body, and spirit.

☐ I've expressed my gratitude for today and all it brings, good and bad.

☐ I've prepared for tomorrow and all the unknowns it might bring.

Day 31 and Beyond

NOW THAT YOU'VE completed these precious 30 days, it's time to reflect on your progress.

What goals have you attained? Have you set some new ones?

What bad habits have you broken? What positive new lifestyle patterns and habits are emerging in your life now? Do you have a healthy obsession?

If you still have some goals to reach or some habits to break, remember this: You now have some skills, strategies, and hopefully tons of inspiration to make it happen. Put down on paper three challenges you are facing right now and brainstorm constructive solutions by drawing from what you learned here. Be the solution to any problems you have.

If there's a stubborn habit that still bothers you, go at it a day at a time. I don't know about you, but I'm not wired to manage long lengths of time. However, I can definitely manage one day at a time. I believe that living one day a time is really the secret of healthy living.

When you get up, be thankful for the day, and begin with a healthy breakfast. From the time you wake up until bedtime, make a conscious effort to be fully engaged in living and enjoying those hours. And finally:

Count your blessings, not calories.

Get active. Physical activity will blast away any trouble, worry, or stress faster than you can say *badass*.

Be kind to yourself—in thoughts and actions.

Know your strengths and put them to work.

Spend time in stillness.

Let go of your stuff.

Avoid negative thoughts and negative influences.

Don't go out of bounds.

Laugh often and much.

Connect with those you love and those who love you.

Live your purpose and your legacy.

Get excited about what will happen if you do all these things.

See you in the badass lane!

30 More Mind-Body-Spirit Challenges for Every Day of the Month

I HOPE MY 30-day program got you fired up and on the right track to success. If you enjoyed it as much as I enjoyed creating it for you, here's a bonus for you: some additional challenges you can try for the next 30 days, if you desire. So dive in, dig deeper, and have fun!

MIND CHALLENGES

Challenge 1. Do visual goal setting.

When you began setting goals on Day 1, those goals may have felt a little shapeless. Here's a solution to complement your goal setting and help you crystallize your goals in a visual way: Construct a *vision board*.

This is basically a collage of pictures that represent your goals. You paste the pictures on a piece of poster board and place the board in an area where you'll, see it all the time. A vision board can enhance your goal-achieving process. Whenever you look at it, you'll feel strong positive feelings of happiness, and these emotions in turn will enhance your desire and motivation to achieve those goals.

To begin, collect and cut out relevant images from magazines or Internet printouts that illustrate your goals. Glue them to your poster board. If your goal is to lose 25 pounds, don't just have a picture of a thin, fit body up there; also include images of how a thin, fit person enjoys life—splashing at the beach, enjoying adventure travels, wearing cute clothes, interacting with people, and so forth. Or if there's something you want in the near future, like a home of your own, create a vision board that reflects your "dream house." A vision board can be created for any goal or collection of goals. Place your board where you can see it daily.

Challenge 2. Talk yourself out of bad habits.

Inner conversations have a powerful effect on your motivation and well-being. What you think determines what you say, how you feel, and how you act. The more affirming your self-talk, the more successful you'll be at booting out bad habits. You can slip out of self-defeating thoughts by making a list of typical negative messages, or "loser statements," and replacing those statements with flip-side positive messages, or "winner statements." Here are some examples:

Loser Statement	Winner Statement
I can't change.	I can change any bad habit when I put my mind to it.
I've tried and I always fail.	I don't always fail. Every positive choice I make is a major success.
I'm not athletic.	Regular exercise makes me feel like an athlete.

In this challenge, replace your loser statements with winner statements. This challenge helps you reshape your thought patterns and pull your out of the negative self-talk rut.

My Loser Statements	My Winner Statements
_____	_____
_____	_____
_____	_____
_____	_____
_____	_____

Challenge 3. Get out of your mental slump.

I've had quite a few people reach out to me in search of advice on battling depression. I'm not talking about the clinically depressed, who require medical and psychological treatment, but rather those feel sad, stuck in a slump from time to time.

If this ever happens to you, work through the following challenge:

Step 1. Dream.

Journal five new things you would like to happen in your life, in the next week or month.

1. _____

2. _____

3. _____

4. _____

5. _____

Step 2. Make it happen.

What's it going to take to make these dreams come true? Save a certain amount of money each week? Revamp some lifestyle issues, such as diet or exercise? Take a course or seminar?

From your list, develop strategies that will manifest these things in your life.

1. _____

2. _____

3. _____

4. _____

5. _____

Step 3. Attract them!

At night before you go to sleep, visualize yourself already having these things. Create the picture, feel it, and hold it intently in your mind. These visualizations, combined with your feelings, function like a magnet. This magnet attracts experiences that match your thoughts and feelings, so if you want something really badly and keep concentrating on it, you increases your changes of obtaining it.

Challenge 4. Enjoy a chuckle.

Laughter serves a protective psychological function by distracting us from the negative side of a situation (like a failure). My challenge for you is start making a humor notebook. Whenever you come across a joke, saying, story, cartoon, or poem that tickles your funny bone, write it down or paste it into your notebook. That way you have access to funny stuff when you need a lift. There's a health and fitness benefit here, too: People who can laugh at themselves and can see humor in everyday occurrences experience less pain, feel healthier, and generally have stronger immune systems.

Challenge 5. Make smarter decisions.

Should you switch careers? Take a new job? Get married? Break up with someone? Buy a house? Sink money into an investment? Go back to school? Change your diet?

Decisions, decisions, decisions. We're faced with them every day. Sometimes we make seat-of-our-pants decisions without considering the consequences. Or we do the opposite. We stall instead of making a decision, letting opportunities slip away.

No matter what the current state of your decision-making habits, you can reprogram your mind to make better choices, most of the time, in every area of your life—personal, professional, and financial. Here's a three-part challenge you can use any time to help you.

Step 1. Research.

Go on a fact-finding mission to learn as much as you can about the choice you are facing. Got a hot tip on a stock investment? Research the company, its performance, its long-term forecast, and all that. Thinking about taking a course? Check it out. Will this course give you all the extra training you really need? Does it result in any sort of certification? Who is the instructor? If you want to switch to a vegetarian diet, learn all the pros and cons and find out how it will work in your lifestyle. Use all available resources on your fact-finding mission: the Internet, books, mentors, and others.

In the spaces below, write down the decision you're facing and what sort of homework is required.

_____

_____

_____

Step 2. Evaluate the situation against your long-term goals.

Ideally, the decisions we make are stepping-stones toward our goals. When faced with a decision, ask yourself if the choice you're about to make will help you meet your goals or send you on a path away from those goals. Think about the following:

Review the goals you set for yourself on day 1. Which goal does the decision you're facing align with?

_____

_____

_____

Will your decision help you reach that goal? Why or why not?

_____

_____

_____

Step 3. Weigh the pros and cons.

Take out a blank sheet of paper. With a pen or pencil (or in your word-processing program), divide the paper into two columns. At the top of the left column, write *Pros*; at the top of the right column, write *Cons*. Then list the advantages and disadvantages of each course of action in the appropriate column.

Some decisions involve moral and ethical issues (such as, "Should I tell my best friend her husband is cheating on her or should I keep my mouth shut?"). In those cases, you may have to weigh your options according to your personal moral, ethical, or spiritual values.

Finally, I think it's a good idea to sleep on your decision. That $3,000 stock tip might not look so desirable tomorrow.

Challenge 6. Quiz: Are You an Emotional Eater?

Read through the following statements. If a statement is true for you a lot the time, circle it. Count up the number of statements you've circled.

1. During stressful times, I tend to engage in unhealthy behaviors (such as eating junk food, binge drinking, or doing harmful drugs).

2. I tend to eat when I'm not hungry, rather than when my body needs nourishment.

3. I feel guilty or ashamed of myself when I overeat.

4. I eat healthy when I'm around others but overeat or binge on unhealthy foods when I'm alone.

5. My overeating (or binge drinking or taking harmful drugs) interferes with my life.

6. I am overweight, but I overeat anyway.

7. My eating behaviors make me unhappy.

8. Being in a bad mood or feeling depressed makes me overeat (or engage in some other bad habit).

9. I spend a lot of time thinking about food or other bad habits.

10. I self-medicate with sugary foods.

SCORING

If you circled five or more questions: You are probably an emotional eater, and situations and moods trigger you to overeat or resort to other bad habits to cope. I would suggest that you seek professional help, because eating to excess may be an attempt to deal with your feelings about something off in your life: loneliness, financial troubles, job problems, or setbacks. Also, read my strategies in the next challenge.

If you circled three or four questions: You might be struggling with a little emotional overeating. I'd say you are borderline. That's not all bad. You can get your eating under control and on a healthy track. Also, read my strategies in the next challenge.

If you circled to two or fewer questions: Don't worry. You're not an emotional overeater. Sure, you might grab a little junk food now and then to deal with stress, but it doesn't interfere with your life or health.

Challenge 7. Don't pull those triggers!

Bad habits can be triggered by people, places, and pressures, all threatening to push us off the wagon with a big thud. The power of people, for instance, is forceful but subtle. Your mom might tempt you with her blasted brownies or those deadly cookies; a business associate might say, "One little drink won't hurt you"; or your best friend might offer you a cigarette.

Locales like your favorite restaurant or that fried chicken joint you drive by on

your way home from work—these can be triggers associated with eating or drinking (too much) alcohol.

Then of course there are life pressures. When you're overwhelmed, it's easy to
go into an unhealthy default mode to soothe yourself with food, alcohol, drugs, or
some other unhealthy habit.

To free yourself from these unhealthy cycles, you must first identify the people,
places, and pressures that trigger your loss of self-control. Here is a work sheet to
help you map out appropriate strategies:

My Personal Triggers	My Strategies for Self-Control
PEOPLE	STRATEGY
Example: Certain friends who love to eat out and are overweight who practice healthy lifestyles	Cultivate a circle of other friends who practice healthy lifestyles.
PLACES	STRATEGY
Example: Snacking or over-snacking	Set a boundary that you will eat food only in your dining room, not in front of the television.
PRESSURES	STRATEGY
Example: I eat when I'm depressed, lonely, bored.	I will distract myself with a nonfood activity such as working out, reading a book, or immersing myself in a hobby.

Challenge 8. Get sharp and focused in an instant.

Sitting at your desk and can't think straight? Then sit up straight.

A slouched, hunched-over sitting position cuts down on the blood flow to your
brain. This is a chief cause of foggy thinking, poor problem solving, and forget-

fulness. Your brain requires nearly thirty times more blood and oxygen than your other organs, so it needs a healthy blood supply in order to function properly.

Poor posture crimps the two arteries that pass through your spine to your brain and reduces blood flow—much like a crimp in a garden hose cuts off water flow. This hinders thinking, memory performance, and other brain skills.

So sit up straight! Imagine that there's a string connecting your skull to the bones in your pelvis. "Pull" that string tight by sitting as straight as you can, with an erect back. You'll feel noticeably more alert and focused in an instant.

Challenge 9. Get creative fast.

Creativity is often elusive—hard to find when you need it the most. I've found a scientifically valid solution that will blow your mind and bring your creativity to greater heights. A study published in the journal *Brain and Cognition* demonstrated that when you strengthen the level of communication between the right and left hemispheres of the brain, you goose up your creativity.

For background: your left hemisphere controls speech and language and deals with logic. It helps you do things in a particular sequence, such as tying your shoes or backing your car out of the driveway. The right side deals with emotion, intuition, creativity visual skills, and spatial abilities. If you were redecorating your house, for example, you'd picture the decor in your head with the right hemisphere of your brain. The left side keeps tabs on the broad thinking of the right, so when both are in sync, you come up with supercreative yet practical ideas.

Back to the study: Sixty-two volunteers performed a creativity task in which they had to come up with as many alternative uses for simple items like paper clips, pencils, and shoes as they could. They were given a minute to do so.

After this task, the researchers asked the volunteers to move their eyes horizontally left to right for thirty seconds, following a target as it moved. A control group was told to just stare ahead.

What happened next was pretty cool. The volunteers repeated the creative task again. Those who had moved their eyes came up with significantly more uses for the objects than the control group did. Why? The researchers pointed out that this exercise increases cross-linking and communications between the two sides of the brain.

Try this challenge yourself! Give yourself a minute to brainstorm as many non-standard uses for a coffee mug (besides as a drink holder) as you can. Make sure these are uncommon. Write down your answers.

Next, move your eyes horizontally from left to right for thirty seconds. Repeat the exercise and see if you can come up with additional uses for the mug.

For practical use, try bilateral eye movement when you've got to solve a problem, you've hit writer's block, or you need to come up with a creative idea for a birthday present. By increasing the interaction between the left and right sides of your brain, you may increase your creative options and solutions.

Challenge 10. Pre-prepare!

With this final mind challenge, welcome to my class in advanced mental toughness. We tend to think of mental toughness in reference to how well you manage stress and react to bad situations. Being mentally tough, however, doesn't mean that you don't cry, get sad or edgy, or just feel crappy. No way! But it does mean that you can deal with this shit and move on. In this challenge, I'd like you to journal how you'd positively deal with and respond to life-changing events. This challenge will help prepare your mind to deal with adversity. In your journal, answer the following:

- How would you react and manage if you were involved in a serious accident or experienced a natural disaster?
- How would you cope if someone very close to you died? (If you have dealt with this before, write down how you'd deal with it differently—or if you dealt with it in a strong way, recall your experience.)
- What plan do you have in place to deal with a lengthy illness or disability?
- How would you manage any unforeseen setbacks, changes, or job loss in your professional career? Consider mental, physical, and spiritual coping strategies.

I know this stuff isn't the greatest material to think about now, but it does force you to give thought to how you'd manage successfully through a crisis before one actually develops.

BODY CHALLENGES

Challenge 1. Break this habit now.

One insidious habit many people have is an addiction to sugar. Sugar addiction is real. Research has demonstrated that eating excess sugar triggers the manufacture of natural opiates in the brain the same way repeated doses of morphine do!

Sugar is bad news. It's really worse than too much dietary fat, because it creates all sorts of metabolic havoc in your body, from blood sugar disturbances (which can make you moody) to obesity. When you eat sugar and sugar-containing junk, your body uses it as energy, rather than tapping into fat stores for fuel. You're sabotaging your own fat-burning efforts. It doesn't take a lot of sugar to do this. Even a small piece of chocolate will upset the fat-burning process and be turned right into body fat. I'm talking about all kinds of sugar, not just the white stuff. Avoid the following for now: table sugar, syrups, honey, molasses, brown sugar, jams, jellies, candy, desserts, ice cream, and baked goods—anything you'd classify as a "sweet" is on the blacklist.

With this challenge, I'd like you to be honest with yourself. Are you a sugar addict? Take the short quiz on page 271 to find out.

Challenge 2. Improve your body image.

The way you think and feel about your appearance is your body image. If you're like many people, your body image is constantly under attack—mostly by you. Somehow you're never quite content with your looks, your size, or your shape. Or you compare your body to the bodies of others, and yours falls short. This attitude spills over into other areas of your life, and you can feel pretty miserable.

This challenge will help you love your body:

Quiz: Could You Be a Sugarholic?

Read through the following questions and circle yes or no after each one.

1. Do you usually eat refined sugar (table sugar, candy, or sweets) most days of the week?

   A. Yes
   B. No

2. Does the thought of giving up sugar make you uneasy, anxious, or sad?

   A. Yes
   B. No

3. Do you reach for sugar or sugary foods when you're stressed out or depressed?

   A. Yes
   B. No

4. Do you keep a lot of sugary foods around your house?

   A. Yes
   B. No

5. Have you tried but failed to cut back on the amount of sugar you eat?

   A. Yes
   B. No

6. Do you feel guilty after eating a lot of sugary foods?

   A. Yes
   B. No

7. Have you ever gone out of your way—like driving to a convenience store late at night—to buy sugary snacks?

   A. Yes
   B. No

8. After you eat too much sugary food, does your energy drop a couple of hours later?

   A. Yes
   B. No

9. Does eating sugar ever make you feel euphoric?

   A. Yes
   B. No

10. Have you ever lied about your sugar intake?

   A. Yes
   B. No

(cont.)

SCORING

Each question represents a symptom of sugar addiction. If you answered yes to four or more questions, there's a good chance that you're hooked on sugar, or on your way to getting hooked.

Here are some steps to help you break your sugar habit:

1. Each day, promise yourself that you will eat no sugar—not in your coffee or tea, no desserts or candy, no sodas or commercial juices, nothing with sugar in it. This might be one of your physical goals each day. The less sugar you eat, the less sugar you'll crave.

2. Eat three full meals daily, with two or three snacks in between. Meals and snacks should include lean proteins, vegetables, and fruit. Eating multiple meals throughout the day helps prevent cravings for sugary foods.

3. Stay hydrated. Feeling hungry for sugar sometimes means you're dehydrated. Drinking enough water—8 to 10 glasses daily—can help fight sugar cravings.

4. Detox your home by removing all sugary junk food. Have veggies and fruit on hand for when sugar cravings hit.

5. Be mindful about your food choices, especially when you are stressed or depressed. Choose healthy foods during these times; sugary foods will only make you feel worse.

6. Stay active. Regular exercise improves your insulin sensitivity, meaning that your body will metabolize any residual sugar more effectively. Exercise also boosts your mood and relieves stress, so that you're less likely to grab sugary snacks.

Create a special photo album of yourself. Fill it with your most flattering pictures. Add to it frequently. Seeing proof that you're gorgeous, despite what your mind tells you, will make you feel great about yourself. It's your evidence that your body is attractive and desirable.

Another challenge: Get naked. Spend 5 minutes admiring your body in the mirror—naked. Now list five things you love or enjoy about your naked body.

_____

_____

_____

_____

_____

Challenge 3. Reclaim your workout schedule.

If you feel like your time for exercising has shrunk, try this challenge.

Split up your workout time: Take in a 20-minute walk prior to work; then walk an extra 20 minutes during your lunch hour or after dinner.

Also, do shorter but more intense workouts. A Canadian study looked into how efficient and effective a 10-minute workout could be compared with the traditional 50-minute routine. For the 10-minute workout, researchers designed three very intense 20-second bouts of all-out, balls-to-the-wall exercise, followed by brief rest periods. After the experimental period of three months, both the short bouts and the standard longer workout produced the exact same improvements in heart function and blood sugar control, even though one workout was longer than the other. So basically, if you can go hard and fast, you can get away with 10 minutes of exercise.

One other strategy if you feel like you have no time for the gym: Set up a small workout room at home and equip it with a few dumbbells, barbells, a stability ball, resistance bands, and an exercise mat. That's all you need for a real badass workout.

Challenge 4. Apply intention-setting to your workout.

When working out, do you just go through the motions?

If so, I challenge you to work out with intention. You'll get better results and enjoy your workout more. Here goes:

Do some strength-training exercises, with weight or your own body. Perform the exercises very slowly and use yoga-like breathing—slow inhales through your nose and exhales through your mouth. (No rushing through the workout like so many of us tend to do!) Set your intention to feel every muscle as you lift and flex. Know that when you put your mind to your workout, you can push yourself to amazing limits. That's the power of setting your intention.

Challenge 5. Stop food boredom.

Sometimes we get bored eating the same old food every day. Here's a challenge to break you out of this rut: Do a salad swap! Have five friends bring a salad in a jar, layered like this: salad dressing, veggies, protein, lettuce, and nuts or cheese. Then exchange and enjoy your salads and new salad recipes. Do this every week to keep the swap going.

Challenge 6. Detox!

Everyone will be coming to this book with different requirements and different habits that need breaking. If you're working on a serious addictive habit such as alcohol or drug abuse or smoking, it's vital to support the withdrawal process with proper nutrition. Prolonged substance abuse or dependency screws up your health by destroying nutrients and preventing their absorption. In large amounts, for example, alcohol flushes many nutrients from the body: thiamine, vitamin B6, and calcium, among others. Smoking robs the body of vital disease-fighting antioxidants.

So my challenge to you is to make sure you're correcting these problems by eating clean: fresh vegetables and fruits, lean proteins, whole grains, good fats, and so on. I'd also suggest that you add some nutritional supplements to your diet: B complex vitamins and milk thistle to restore liver health; calcium and magnesium for their calming benefits, and vitamin C for detoxification. Start taking these today!

Challenge 7. Get over food guilt.

Feeling guilty over eating certain foods gives food control over you and is a bad habit itself. Here is a challenge that will help empower you:

- Select a "nondiet food" such as a cupcake, a candy bar, a bowl of fancy ice cream, a small bag of chips, and so forth. But do this only if you want to try this challenge!
- Eat it slowly, with no distractions. Savor each bite.
- After you enjoyed your treat, how did you feel? Satisfied? (Great!) Guilty? (Not so great!) If this exercise sent you on a little guilt trip, we need to talk.
- Put a few more foods on your okay-to-eat-as-a-treat list. Let yourself sample some of these regularly.

Scared you'll dive into a gallon of ice cream and hit the bottom of the carton? Some good news: The chances are firmly against it. Nutritionists say that when you allow yourself to eat certain foods, the desire to eat them in large quantities eventually goes away. This challenge will help you stop obsessing over everything you put in your mouth, and stop feeling guilty for eating what you love. You'll be in control of food, not the other way around.

Challenge 8. Ease body tension quickly.

One of the first signs of stress is that your muscles tense up, and you can physically feel anxiety. Head physical stress off at the pass like this:

Sit in a quiet place and begin to take deep breaths. As you do so, drop your tongue from the roof of your mouth. This simple action relaxes your tongue, then your jaw, and finally your neck and shoulders—a real domino effect that can move you from physical stress to relaxation and calm.

Challenge 9. Make a tiny change.

I have talked often throughout this book about the importance of trying new things—"changing the scenery," as I call it. Maybe change still scares you a bit. If so, I have a challenge to help you: make a small change that will benefit your body.

Try a new form of exercising today: a different class at your gym, or on television or YouTube, or using a DVD. Do it just for today. How did it go? How did it make you feel? Would you do it again and why? Record your answers below or in your journal.

Challenge 10. Plan an active vacation.

I love having something to look forward to, such as a great vacation. The prospect of taking off and doing something fun lifts my spirits and keeps me in a great mood. For a lot of us, vacation means relaxation—lying in the sun on a beach, napping poolside, and eating at great restaurants. And sure, sometimes this is exactly what you need to recharge.

This year, why not plan an active vacation? Here are some examples:

- A fitness-spa weekend
- A yoga retreat
- A family fitness cruise
- Hiking
- Biking
- Backpacking and camping
- Ranching and horseback riding
- Kayaking, stand-up paddleboarding, or surfing
- Sports or strength camps

So my challenge to you is: Talk to a travel agency, access Expedia or Travelocity, or google various types of active vacations. Then book one!

SPIRITUAL CHALLENGES

Challenge 1. Find quotable quotes.

Using quote books or Internet sites, research quotes from famous people. Write down the ones that inspire you and touch your heart. Keep them handy as affirmations. Work on memorizing them to make them part of you.

Record five of your favorite quotes in the space here:

_____

_____

_____

_____

_____

Challenge 2. Eat mindfully.

There is mindful eating, and there is mindless eating. Mindless eating is a major contributor to obesity; it means wolfing down food, without paying attention to what you're eating because you're watching TV or fiddling with your cell phone. Mindful eating, on the other hand, means focusing on each bite of food, eating slowly, and eliminating mealtime distractions. It prevents autopilot eating—popping food into your mouth without any awareness as to what you're eating or how much.

When you eat mindfully and slowly, your brain is allowed to register that you're full, so you'll feel more satisfied. Plus, you'll keep your weight under better control. In a study published in the journal *Complementary Therapies in Medicine*, volunteers reported much less hunger after six weeks of mindful eating. And in a study at Texas Christian University, people who spent 22 minutes eating their meals consumed 88 fewer calories than those who wolfed down their meals in 9 minutes.

Here is a challenge to help you eat more mindfully:

Do not shovel down your treat while reading a magazine, working on the computer, or watching TV. Eat it slowly; your goal isn't to finish it as fast as possible. Pay attention to the color, smell, flavor, and texture of the food, chewing slowly and avoiding distractions. If it's a dessert, enjoy it with a nice cup of tea or coffee (great for dunking). Try to make it look and taste as appealing as possible—use a pretty plate or cup, for example.

Challenge 3. Be thankful for your food.

As you prepare, cook, and eat your meals, be thankful for the food. Remind yourself that enjoying fresh, healthy meals instead of processed food is an act of love toward yourself and those you cook for.

Challenge 4. Forgive to live successfully.

People do things to us, and we to them. They may lie to us, betray us, or hurt us—and vice versa. After being hurt, we have a choice: Carry the pain in our hearts or let it go. Holding the pain in, many experts believe, leads to unhappiness and depression, and harms the immune system, leaving you vulnerable to scary diseases. An unforgiving spirit can thus be physically and mentally destructive.

Let go of past hurts and forgive others. You don't even have to do it face-to-face; do it in your heart. Forgiveness is a spiritual act that you do for yourself.

Challenge 5. Spend an hour in silence.

Take a lesson from the monastic life: practice silence—but for only an hour a day. You'll be surprised at what happens. External noise goes away first, and then inner noise starts to fade. Soon quiet envelops you, it seems. Time slows down. You might hear only natural sounds, the patter of rain on a window, the wind blowing through trees, or birds chirping—all sounds that lead to further inner calm.

Here's how to carry out this challenge:

- Decide on, and schedule, your hour of silence at a certain time each day.
- Turn off the television, computer, phone, and any machine or appliance that generates noise. Avoid any written communication, unless it's an inspirational article or book.
- Light a candle as a spiritual symbol to your hour of silence.
- Sit quietly and rest, or move around slowly.
- Listen to the silence and stay in the present moment. Notice how much more calm you feel.
- Breathe deeply and mindfully, inhaling the silence and exhaling the internal "noise."
- At the end of silent hour, let your first word be an expression of thanks, gratitude, or love. Extinguish your candle, and go about the rest of your day, refreshed and calm.

Challenge 6. Write "morning pages."

Here's a little spiritual secret I picked up from a friend: Grab a notebook and write down "life" questions shortly after you get up in the morning. Don't be surprised if something quite "otherworldly" happens.

For example, pose a question that has been bugging you and write it down, such as "What should I do about my debt?" Then just listen; you might hear wisdom coming from somewhere beyond yourself, like "Keep track of the money coming in and going out" or "Now's the time to turn that hobby into profit." Or maybe you write: "What can I do about my spouse's negativity?" An answer comes back: "Forgive him" or "Have a respectful dialogue with him about my feelings."

Morning pages are not like journaling, in which you explore personal issues in depth. Instead, they're like spiritual radar that transmits messages back and forth from whatever or whoever you call your higher power, or even your own intuition. Do this consistently, and you'll get rid of negative debris in your psyche and open up spiritual channels. Give it a chance!

Challenge 7. Dig in your garden.

I know a lot of people who garden. Many grow their own vegetables, for example, because they want to avoid pesticides, soil contaminants, and other health hazards. Others claim gardening is a stress reliever because it's fun and active. Still others describe gardening as a spiritual activity that connects them with nature. What's not to love about gardening?

If you have a yard or garden, take time this week to tend it—and you'll discover that you're also tending your mind, body, and soul.

No yard? Try growing herbs in pots placed near a window for sunlight. Herb gardening can be very healing, both in the physical and spiritual sense. Feverfew, for example, empowers the immune system. Basil can ease the symptoms of digestive problems. So can peppermint. Tea prepared from the flowers of chamomile is believed to be a moderate sedative. All of these herbs can be easily grown in pots or outdoors.

So why not try something new? Grow a medicinal herb garden!

Challenge 8. Engage with a spiritual text.

Throughout this book, I've said that reading spiritual and inspirational texts is a wonderful way to enhance your spirituality. But with this challenge, I want to dig a little deeper and help you get the most from these texts.

There are four ways to interact with a spiritual text: read, reflect, respond, and rest. First, read the passage or chapter slowly. Second, stop and ask yourself: "What is this passage saying?" Third, read it again, and ask: "What is this passage saying *to me*?"

Finally, if you respond to the passage with positive feelings—say, an insight, a feeling of gratitude, or the realization of an action you must take—then reflect on how to act upon its wisdom and apply it to your life.

Challenge 9. Go high tech for high spirituality.

Spirituality doesn't come easily to everyone. Sometimes you need a gentle nudge to journal, meditate, pray, or spend some quiet time.

Apps to your rescue! There are many spiritual apps you can download. Some provide guided breathing exercises to produce inner calm and ease anxiety. Others provided guided meditations. Many apps provide prayers and other spiritual practices.

Get started on this challenge by googling "spiritual apps." There's something out there for everyone.

Challenge 10. Thank your bad habits.

You've been working on ridding your life of habits that have stood in the way of your happiness and success. You may not realize it yet, but those bad habits came with some powerful lessons. Perhaps you've learned how to improve your finances, get healthier and happier, or stop making poor choices. Right now, be thankful for that learning and experience. Thank your bad habits for being the catalyst that got you out of the dark and into the light.

References

Dai, C. L., and M. Sharma. 2014. Between inhale and exhale: yoga as an intervention in smoking cessation. *Journal of Evidence-Based Complementary & Alternative Medicine* 19(2): 144–149.

Daly, P., et al. 2016. A mindful eating intervention: A theory-guided randomized anti-obesity feasibility study with adolescent Latino females. *Complementary Therapies in Medicine* 28: 22–28.

Dartigues, J. F. 2013. Playing board games, cognitive decline and dementia: a French population-based cohort study. *BMJ Open* 3(8); doi:10.1136/bmjopen-2013–002998.

Denham, J., et al. 2016. Increased expression of telomere-regulating genes in endurance athletes with long leukocyte telomeres. *Journal of Applied Physiology* 120(2): 148–158.

Epton, T., and P. R. Harris. 2008. Self-affirmation promotes health behavior change. *Health Psychology* 27(6): 746–752.

Ferrin, L. 2009. Yosemite's rock stars. *The Atlantic*, May, online.

Gillen, J. B., et al. 2016. Twelve weeks of sprint interval training improves indices of cardiometabolic health similar to traditional endurance training despite a five-fold lower exercise volume and time commitment. *PLOS ONE*, April 26; dx.doi.org/10.1371/journal-pone.0154075.

Hallgren, M., et al. 2014. Yoga as an adjunct treatment for alcohol dependence: a pilot study. *Complementary Therapies in Medicine* 22(3): 441–445.

Miyake, A., et al. 2010. Reducing the gender achievement gap in college science: a classroom study of values affirmation. *Science* 330(6008): 1234–1237.

Newberg, A. B., et al. 2014. Meditation and neurodegenerative diseases. *Annals of the New York Academy of Sciences* 1307: 112–123.

Oppezzo, M., and D. L. Schwartz. 2014 Give your ideas some legs: The positive effect of walking on creative thinking. *Journal of Experimental Psychology: Learning, Memory, and Cognition* 40(4): 1142–1152.

Phillips-Caesar, E. G., et al. 2015. Small Changes and Lasting Effects (SCALE) Trial: the formation of a weight loss behavioral intervention using EVOLVE. *Contemporary Clinical Trials* 41: 118–128.

Rahe, R., et al. 1964. Social stress and illness onset. *Journal of Psychosomatic Research* 8(1): 35–44.

Saxbe, D. E., and R. Repetti. 2010. No place like home: home tours correlate with daily patterns of mood and cortisol. *Personality & Social Psychology Bulletin* 36(1): 71–81.

Shah, M., et al. 2014. Slower eating speed lowers energy intake in normal-weight but not overweight/obese subjects. *Journal of the Academy of Nutrition and Dietetics* 114(3): 393–402.

Shortland, G. 2014. Back on the board: Bethany Hamilton lost a limb in a shark attack but, remarkably, she was back in the sea and riding to success just weeks later. *The People,* May 18, online.

Shobe, E. R., et al. 2009. Influence of handedness and bilateral eye movements on creativity. *Brain and Cognition* 71(3): 204–214.

Stringfellow, J. 2013. 60 affirmations to support you through meaningful life changes. *Spirituality & Health*, January–February, online.

Tucker, L. A., and K. Maxwell. 1992. Effects of weight training on the emotional well-being and body image of females: predictors of greatest benefit. *American Journal of Health Promotion* 6(5): 338–344.

Vidoni, E. D. 2015. Dose-response of aerobic exercise on cognition: A community-based, pilot randomized controlled trial. *PLOS ONE*, July 9: dx.doi.org/10.1371/journalpone.013167.

Acknowledgments

I would like to express my deepest appreciation and gratitude to my publisher, William Morrow/HarperCollins; my editor, Cassie Jones; my book agent, Steve Troha; my cowriter, Maggie Greenwood-Robinson; my right-hand woman, Jenny Armour; and Holly Mendenhall, my NYC muse and editor. Without each of you, this book would still be roaming around inside my head and heart. Thank you to you and your teams for coming together and helping this book become a reality; I appreciate all the time, effort, and endless hours that you put into this project with me. I feel deeply fortunate that I have such a skilled and passionate team beside me.

I would also like to thank all the servicepersons and veterans out there who have served selflessly for my freedom to write this book and live an exceptional life. There's not a day that I do not give thanks for your service and all that each of you do. I hope to continue to support you in every way I can through my own services and efforts to honor you and our country.

Furthermore, I would like to thank Chazz, Ray, and Brandon . . . no last names needed here. Each of you played a different role as a huge contributor to finding and owning my mental tenacity—my "baby monster"—throughout this journey. Thank you for not treating me any less than what you knew I could be.

Thank you to my photographers, Rick Elder (aka "The Warden"), Tyler Northup, and Paul Bucceta, who worked very hard on a tight schedule to make beautiful photos for this book. You each have a different eye and skill, but somehow they all come together to yield my best work yet. Thank you for putting up with so much and always seeing the magic that I was trying to create.

Thank you to *all* my fans for your continued support as you've grown with me. This has been an incredible journey, and I hope to continue to inspire each one of you daily. Thank you for helping me share my experiences to a wider audience and help the world.

Oh, dear family! Thank you for knowing I was different and embracing me as I was. You've all been part of my personal journey, which made this book what it is. Mom, thank you for encouraging me to go to Iraq so many years ago. Your daring to save me is what started this new life and journey. As always, you are my hero. Kole, you have continued to amaze me with your refusal to conform to anything but what you want. Thank you for being such a great role model, early on and now. Chris, you and I are so similar it's dangerous. Thank you for showing me that you can always be kind and help someone in need. Dad, you are a rolling stone through and through! Thank you for showing me what hard work looks like and always following your heart. John, I know you always have my back and will always be down to throw down! I am proud to be your family.

I can't close without giving acknowledgment and gratitude to my best friend and partner. Geoff, you saw me work through this process from start to end. Thank you for always believing in my ability do anything I put my mind to, and to change the world in the process. Your constant belief in my potential and ability still gives me flutters. Here's to many more years of going in headfirst—and knowing the best is yet to come!

Index